Cognitive-Behavioral Therapy with Black Americans

Virgil L. Gregory, Jr.

Cognitive-Behavioral Therapy with Black Americans

A Principle and Structurally Informed Perspective

Springer

Virgil L. Gregory, Jr.
School of Social Work
Indiana University
Indianapolis, IN, USA

ISBN 978-3-032-01665-2 ISBN 978-3-032-01666-9 (eBook)
https://doi.org/10.1007/978-3-032-01666-9

This Springer imprint is published by the registered company Springer Nature Switzerland AG
The registered company address is: Gewerbestrasse 11, 6330 Cham, Switzerland

The author wishes to dedicate this work to his late father, Virgil L. Gregory, Sr.

Preface

The last several decades have seen cognitive-behavioral therapy (CBT) advanced in both science and practice. Research supporting cognitive models and cognitive-behavioral interventions for various psychiatric disorders continues to be published. The adoption of cognitive-behavioral interventions by a vast array of helping professionals remains strong and continues to grow.

Despite the empirical and practical advances of CBT, CBT for Black Americans has not experienced the same growth in practice. Despite this fact, clinically relevant research that advances cognitive-behavioral practice for Black Americans exists. The extant and emerging cognitive-behavioral research includes traditional targets of cognitive-behavioral interventions such as thoughts and behaviors as well as structural factors that may complicate the delivery of cognitive-behavioral interventions with Black American clients.

The cognitive-behavioral literature currently lacks a coherent and research-based framework for identifying and explaining key modifiable aspects of CBT with Black Americans, in the context of long-standing structural racism. The present text, *Cognitive-Behavioral Therapy with Black Americans: A Principle and Structurally Informed Perspective*, provides cognitive-behavioral clinicians with 10 principles. These 10 principles outline fundamental aspects of CBT with Black Americans and provides functional applications for optimizing CBT with Black Americans. The text is divided into three sections.

Part I, Cognitive-Behavioral Therapy with Black Americans: Past and Present, provides historical and structural context of CBT with Black Americans.

Part II, Cognitive-Behavioral Principles and Interventions with Black Americans, addresses theoretical and practical applications of CBT with Black Americans, in the context of anti-Black structural racism. This section addresses the effect of implicit racial bias on CBT with Black Americans as well as the application of the 10 cognitive-behavioral principles for Black Americans, collectively referred to by the acronym RESPPECTUS, Trademark Pending.

Part III, RESPPECTUS Principles: Applications to Black Demographic Groups, addresses the use of CBT and the RESPPECTUS principles with Black Men,

Women, and members of the Black Diaspora in Canada, South Africa, and South America.

The author is grateful to God for the opportunities to work with Black American clients and participants who courageously worked with the author in clinical cognitive-behavioral and community-engaged research settings, respectively.

Indianapolis, IN, USA Virgil L. Gregory Jr.

Competing Interests The author has no competing interests to declare that are relevant to the content of this manuscript.

Contents

About the Author

Virgil L. Gregory Jr., PhD is an associate professor at the Indiana University School of Social Work. Dr. Gregory is a licensed clinical social worker and licensed clinical addictions counselor. Dr. Gregory has clinical experience in using cognitive-behavioral therapy in the treatment of Black Americans and other persons with mood, anxiety, psychotic, and substance use disorders. His research evaluates cognitive-behavioral therapy for substance use disorders, affective disorders, and Black Americans. Dr. Gregory's research has placed specific emphasis on the intersection of Black male mental health and social injustice. As a cognitive-behavioral therapist and researcher, Dr. Gregory's studies include scale development and psychometric evaluation of the aforementioned topic areas. A consistent theme is the translation of research into clinical practice. His research also incorporates systematic reviews, meta-analyses, and clinical trials.

Part I
Cognitive-Behavioral Therapy with Black Americans: Past and Present

Chapter 1
The Historical Context of Cognitive-Behavioral Therapy with Black Americans

1.1 Cognitive-Behavioral Therapy: Theory and Intervention Summary

Cognitive-behavioral theory is premised on the notion that an individual's interpretation of an event is associated with emotional consequences (Beck, 1976). Therefore, if an individual experiences an event and has thoughts of danger, those thoughts about danger contribute to anxious feelings. Similarly, self-devaluating thoughts about an event contribute to feelings of sadness or depression. Cognitive models underscore the relationships among events, thoughts/beliefs, and emotions. Ellis's (1994) activating events, beliefs, consequences, and disputation (ABCD) model suggests that emotions are not directly caused by events but instead are mediated by thoughts/beliefs. That is, an individual does not experience an emotion based solely on an event; an individual experiences an emotion in part due to the thoughts or beliefs the individual has about the event. Ellis maintains that since beliefs (B) about events (A) contribute to emotional and behavioral consequences (C), undesirable emotions and behaviors can be changed by challenging or disputing beliefs that necessitate them (D). Beck's (2021) cognitive model highlights the role of cognition in influencing emotions and behavior; however, Beck proposes a hierarchy of cognitive structures and makes distinctions among different types of beliefs. Cognitive models underscore the importance of changing thoughts/beliefs to change emotions and behaviors.

Since the inception of cognitive-behavioral therapy (CBT) in the 1950s (Beck, 1952), CBT has grown to include an array of interrelated interventions. These psychotherapeutic approaches include cognitive-therapy (Leahy, 1996), cognitive-behavior modification (Meichenbaum, 1977), schema therapy (Young et al., 2003), rational emotive behavior therapy (Ellis, 1994), mindfulness-based cognitive therapy (Segal et al., 2013), acceptance and commitment therapy (Hayes et al., 2012),

V. L. Gregory, Jr., *Cognitive-Behavioral Therapy with Black Americans*,
https://doi.org/10.1007/978-3-032-01666-9_1

dialectical behavior therapy (Linehan, 1993), and others that fit within three waves of CBT interventions over 50 years (Hayes, 2016). While references are made to the first and third waves of CBT throughout the book when relevant, the primary emphasis is on second-wave, Beckian CBT. Cognitive-behavioral therapy is a psychosocial treatment that integrates client characteristics (events, beliefs, thoughts, emotions, behaviors, and positive attributes) to formulate cognitive and behavioral interventions that ameliorate disorder-specific symptoms and achieve client goals (Beck, 2021). Cognitive-behavioral therapy uses a number of strategies including but not limited to the Socratic method (Overholser, 2010) and numerous forms of behavioral treatment (Gambrill, 1994). In accordance with the function and methods of CBT, intervention targets typically include latent constructs like thoughts, beliefs, attributions, meanings, attitudes, and directly observable phenomena like behaviors or relationship functioning. Both the aforementioned cognitive structures and behavior are viewed in the context of the social environment (Granvold, 1994).

1.2 Cognitive-Behavioral Disorder-Specific Models and Treatment Manuals

Many disorder-specific and transdiagnostic models have been theoretically developed and/or empirically evaluated using a cognitive-behavioral framework: depression (Pössel & Black, 2014), anxiety (Ishikawa, 2015), psychosis (Cather et al., 2004), gambling (Raylu et al., 2016), substance use (Beck et al., 1993), transdiagnostic models of eating disorders (Lampard et al., 2013), and anxiety (Norton & Paulus, 2017) among many others. Cognitive-behavioral treatment manuals have also been published to aid in research fidelity and the effective clinical implementation of CBT for depression (Beck et al., 1979), anxiety (Beck et al., 1985), personality disorders (Beck et al., 2015), psychosis (Beck et al., 2009), substance use (Wenzel et al., 2012), eating disorders (Fairburn, 2008), and transdiagnostic treatment of anxiety (Norton, 2012). In addition to the cognitive-behavioral models and disorder-specific treatment manuals for individual therapy, CBT has been manualized in marital (Rathus & Sanderson, 1999) and group (Free, 1999; Sank & Shaffer, 1984) therapy modalities as well. The advancement of cognitive-behavioral models and treatments has been spurred by research evaluating the efficacy of the psychosocial intervention.

1.3 The Meta-Analytic Efficacy of Cognitive-Behavioral Therapy

Cognitive-behavioral therapy is the most researched psychotherapy (David et al., 2018; McMain et al., 2015). The number of primary studies, especially randomized controlled trials (RCTs), evaluating CBT's efficacy in treating various psychiatric disorders and conditions helps facilitate the conduct of meta-analytic studies. For the purpose of the present discussion, a meta-analysis (Glass, 1976) is a quantitative synthesis of independent studies, the results of which allow researchers to determine the overall effect of a particular intervention for a particular disorder. An initial review of CBT meta-analyses showed moderate or large effect sizes for various anxiety disorders, major depressive disorder, posttraumatic stress disorder (PTSD), marital distress, chronic pain, and somatic disorders (Butler et al., 2006). Another review of CBT meta-analyses found the most compelling support for anger, anxiety disorders, bulimia, basic distress, and somatoform disorders (Hofmann et al., 2012). A more recent meta-analytic review of cognitive-behavioral RCTs have demonstrated the efficacy of CBT in improving anxiety, depression, quality of life (QOL), and pain outcomes compared to control groups (Fordham et al., 2021). As it pertains to cognitive-behavioral modalities other than individual therapy, meta-analytic examinations of RCTs have robust findings for CBT's efficacy in treating couples for relationship distress (Gregory, 2021). Cognitive-behavioral group therapy has also been shown to efficaciously treating a number of issues (Johnsen & Thimm, 2018; Koffel et al., 2015). Cognitive-behavioral therapy is considered the gold standard of psychotherapy (David et al., 2018). This finding was based on CBT's outcomes, relative to other psychotherapies, CBT's extant body of clinical research, CBT's lack of comparative inferiority, research supporting CBT models and mechanisms, and the number of clinicians who have adopted a CBT treatment orientation. The overall research supporting CBT's impact on psychiatric diagnoses and different human conditions is quite impressive.

1.4 Cognitive-Behavioral Therapy: Racial Considerations Regarding Black Stakeholders

With CBT's substantial research findings and manualized treatment procedures for clinicians, the question of "What is the status of CBT for Black Americans" becomes more obvious. The term "status" must first be considered, as it could mean several different things, including: 1) What interests or stake do Black Americans have in CBT? 2) How do traditional cognitive-behavioral principles align with Black American issues? 3) How has CBT been used by clinicians who provide the intervention? and 4) What is the efficacy and effectiveness of CBT for Black Americans? These questions are of equal importance for clinicians who work in racially diverse locations where Black clients may be more prevalent and clinicians who may be treating Black Americans who live in predominantly White locations. Clinicians who work routinely with Black clients and clinicians who rarely work with Black clients must be prepared to competently build and maintain therapeutic relationships that are necessary for the use of CBT interventions with Black American clients. The aforementioned questions are not only of importance to clinicians, but clinical researchers conducting studies with Black individuals have a vested interest in the status of CBT for Black Americans. Such clinical researchers may be using community-based participatory research or other forms of community-engaged research, with Black communities to address the impacts of systemic racism and its clinical implications. Beyond clinicians and researchers, the most important stakeholders in CBT therapy for Black clients are the Black clients themselves. Clients generally experience a power imbalance when participating in psychotherapy (Edge & Lemetyinen, 2019). This power imbalance has the potential to be amplified when the client is a cultural minority, and the clinician is a member of the majority culture. Black and other cultural minority clients have the tension of working to have their treatment goals met while simultaneously navigating the racial nuances of communication, diagnosis, treatment planning, and payment.

Family members, be they spouses, children, parents, or even fictive kin, also have an interest in the outcomes of CBT with Black American clients. Black American family members may be particularly interested in whether the individual, identified as a client, has improved symptoms, functioning, or relationships since participating in CBT. Other familial interests may pertain less to the outcomes but more to the identified client's experience itself. For example, was the cognitive-behavioral therapist understanding or culturally responsive to the needs of the Black American client? General systems theory in families (Nichols & Davis, 2017) illustrates the basic mechanisms by which Black clients engaged in CBT or any other therapy may impact the family system for better or worse. Each Black individual participating in CBT does not exist in isolation. Instead, Black individuals are part of multiple systems, including family and community. Individual perceptive and experiential exchanges of information to other systems (family and racial community), regarding CBT, can influence thoughts, beliefs, and ultimately steer racial minority mental healthcare decisions. In summary, both family members and communities of Black clients have an interest in CBT outcomes and processes. Both systems are directly and indirectly linked to the Black client's treatment goals and experiences, which may promote or impede Black community members' engagement in CBT or other mental healthcare.

1.5 The Use of Psychotherapeutic Services by Black Americans

Pertinent to the discussion of CBT among Black clients is the overall use of mental health services by Black Americans (Olfson et al., 2023). In a year's time, Black and Hispanic Americans were just under half as likely as their White counterparts to receive outpatient mental health treatment. As it pertained to gender, fairly similar trends of underutilization of outpatient mental health services could be seen in comparisons between White men and women and their Black and Hispanic counterparts. Black and Hispanic individuals are also less likely to receive treatment for depression and anxiety disorders. However, Black individuals were more likely to receive treatment for trauma and stress-related issues than Whites and Hispanics. The study by Olfson and colleagues found that, for individuals already engaged in outpatient treatment, Black individuals were more likely than both Hispanic and White individuals to receive psychotherapy. Therefore, while buttressing some themes of mental healthcare underutilization among racial minorities, statistics also show some promising findings regarding the use of psychotherapy among Black persons in the United States.

1.6 The Use of Cognitive-Behavioral Therapy with Black Americans: Clinicians and Clients

The use of CBT with Black American clients can be viewed from several perspectives, including the cognitive-behavioral clinicians who provide CBT and the Black clients who receive CBT. Research addressing clinicians' use of CBT with Black clients will be discussed first, then research evaluating Black client user perspectives of CBT will be considered.

1.6.1 Clinician Use of Cognitive-Behavioral Therapy with Black Americans

As CBT evolves, the implementation or actual use of CBT in accordance with the way it was intended (fidelity; Allen et al., 2018) becomes even more relevant. Empirical articles addressing CBT and issues of fidelity with Black participants are limited. However, two independent studies, one experimental (Ezawa & Strunk, 2022a) and the other observational (Ezawa & Strunk, 2022b), examined therapists' preferences for and use of cognitive-behavioral interventions with Black clients. The experimental study examined the therapists' preferences in providing cognitive restructuring or validation with Black versus White hypothetical clients (Ezawa & Strunk, 2022a). In this study 88% of the therapists were White. Therapists were asked about cognitive-behavioral treatment preferences for the hypothetical clients in both arms of the study. The study found therapists thought that validation would be more important than cognitive restructuring for Black individuals. Similarly, the therapists indicated they would spend more time on validation than cognitive restructuring for Black clients. Another study by Ezawa & Strunk (2022b) used preexisting study data on CBT for depression. The purpose of the study was to determine the extent to which therapists working with actual Black and White clients, engaged in cognitive and behavioral methods and the strength of the therapeutic alliance. In the observational study 100% of the therapists were White (Ezawa & Strunk, 2022b). While differences between symptoms and attrition were null, the study did find that therapists used significantly less cognitive methods with Black clients, relative to their White counterparts. In the observational study, the authors acknowledge that cognitive methods in both Black and White patients were equally related to outcome and state that the notion of using cognitive methods less frequently with Black clients was challenged by their results. Ezawa & Strunk (2022a) state that the absence of empirical data suggesting cognitive methods should be used less often with Black clients could indicate a lack of fidelity in the use of CBT with Black clients. Given the clinical complexities that permeate both practice and research regarding CBT for Black Americans, an examination of the Black client user experiences with CBT and the empirical status of CBT for Black Americans is appropriate.

1.6.2 Black Client User Experiences with Cognitive-Behavioral Therapy

The experiences of Black clients and other racial minorities, who have used CBT to address various psychiatric issues, have often been investigated using qualitative research methods. These methods allow for rich, detailed descriptions of client experiences and the exploration of the meaning (Padgett, 2017) attached to experiences with receiving CBT. The research examining Black client experiences with CBT has typically addressed issues of therapeutic rapport, perceptions of providers, the processes, and supposed mechanisms of change in CBT (Gurpinar-Morgan et al., 2014; Rathod et al., 2010). Examinations of Black adolescent user experiences demonstrate the need for cognitive-behavioral clinicians to understand how (Gurpinar-Morgan et al., 2014):

1. Racial factors influence presenting problems.
2. To maximize empathy.
3. Race influences treatment.
4. To adopt a proactive stance in discussing the client's racial background and experiences.
5. To avoid making assumptions when the clinician's race is congruent with the client's race.

Another study (Rathod et al., 2010), also conducted in the United Kingdom, included persons of African descent as well Pakistani and Bangladeshi descent. This study evaluated feedback from clients, lay people, and clinicians regarding CBT interventions for people with psychosis. The key points for cognitive-behavioral clinicians working with Black and other racial minorities included the following:

1. The clinician has the prime responsibility for building and maintaining therapeutic rapport given cynicism that may already be present with racial groups.
2. Problem-solving and mindfulness interventions may be particularly useful.
3. Behaviorally and socially oriented interventions may be more useful at the outset of therapy.

4. The importance of culturally relevant supervision.

Thus far, data describing the use of CBT for Black individuals by clinicians and client experiences with said interventions have been briefly discussed. The empirical outcomes of CBT for Black individuals with psychiatric disorders must be examined to understand CBT's history with Black individuals.

1.7 The Empirical Status of Cognitive-Behavioral Therapy for Black Americans

A consistent theme across different clinical trials and meta-analysis, addressing CBT for Black Americans, is that the research is scant, and more research is needed. For the meta-analyses that address Black participants, these analyses sometimes included primary studies/clinical trials with samples that are not exclusively Black. A previous review of CBT meta-analyses (Hofmann et al., 2012) found that but for a few exceptions, few meta-analyses existed for cultural minorities. This has changed somewhat over the years. Therefore, while it is true that clinical research is lagging regarding empirical examination of CBT's efficacy and effectiveness, it is still beneficial to summarize the extant clinical research in the context of the history of CBT with Black Americans.

1.7.1 Systematic Reviews Examining Race/Ethnicity

Various narrative reviews have evaluated Black-relevant CBT research across a number of diagnostic categories. As it pertains to CBT's efficacy for various psychiatric disorders among Black individuals, the lumping of Black participants with other non-White participants limits the generalizability of such findings to Black clients. The narrative reviews often use vote counting (Borenstein et al., 2021) and have legitimately been critiqued for their lack of statistical precision. The narrative reviews included in this chapter are used to underscore the progressive history of CBT for Black individuals with psychiatric disorders. Overall, in the context of the inherent limitations of a narrative review, the results suggest there is some tentative optimism regarding CBT's potential to be efficaciously used with Black individuals to address various psychiatric issues.

As it pertained to depression, panic disorder with agoraphobia, and substance use, Black-relevant findings were obtained from Horrell's (2008) narrative review of CBT for ethnic minorities. Cognitive-behavioral therapy was suggested as a possibly efficacious treatment for depression; however, issues with attrition were noted. Culturally adapted CBT was suggested as beneficial for Black women and there was a vacuum of clinical information regarding Black men and CBT's efficacy. For panic disorder with agoraphobia, Horrell cited one study supporting the large effect sizes from a culturally adapted CBT. For substance use, Horrell's review found that CBT had some effectiveness in decreasing the amount and occurrence of cocaine and alcohol use with a sample of predominantly Black participants. Similar to the findings of CBT for depression, Horrell also found that attrition was an issue with CBT for substance use treatment. A scoping review for cannabis use with predominantly Black samples found CBT to be effective for decreasing cannabis use in Black youth (Montgomery et al., 2017). The scoping review also demonstrated the effectiveness of motivational enhancement therapy and CBT for cannabis use. Another narrative reviewing evaluating CBT for Black American youth and adolescents found the intervention had positive outcomes regarding aggressive, hyperactive, and disruptive target behaviors (Wilson & Cottone, 2013). The same narrative review identified some studies and positive outcomes with CBT for Black Americans with posttraumatic stress disorder, anxiety disorders, and other emotional and behavioral issues. It should be noted that this narrative review was substantially limited by the inclusion of some samples that were not exclusively Black Americans. Appendix A provides a non-exhaustive list of CBT trials and reviews specific to Black individuals.

1.7.2 Meta-Analyses of Internalized Disorders/Symptoms

There are now several meta-analytic studies that aid in summarizing CBT's quantitative effect in addressing various symptom categories among Black individuals. The cognitive-behavioral meta-analyses regarding CBT for Black individuals can be categorized into internalized (depression and anxiety) and externalized (substance use, impulsivity-oriented issues) symptoms or disorders. In contrast to the previously discussed narrative reviews of CBT for Black individuals, the meta-analyses have more recently been conducted, provide a degree of statistical precision, provide more comprehensive answers to clinical questions, and therefore have greater clinical utility. Although the pool of meta-analytic studies that evaluated CBT for psychiatric symptoms and disorders in Black people is small, overall, the cognitive-behavioral findings have yielded effect sizes that are promising and indicative of benefit. A meta-analysis in Gregory Jr., 2016 (Gregory), showed that CBT had moderate overall effects that favored CBT in the treatment of depressive symptoms with Black adult individuals. In this meta-analysis, a less methodologically rigorous subgroup of studies (pretest–posttest designs) had a larger overall effect size. However, the difference in effect sizes between studies that used pretest–posttest designs and control groups was not statistically significant. The author concluded that the effect size findings were roughly analogous to what has been found in CBT studies of depression that were not limited to Black individuals. Similarly, a meta-analysis examining CBT's effect on anxious symptoms in Black adult persons (Gregory Jr., 2019), found that CBT had a large, favorable, and statistically significant effect on the reduction of anxious symptoms in Black study participants. What was compelling about the CBT meta-analysis on Black individuals with anxiety was that the magnitude of the effect size remained large and statistically significant regardless of the categorical methodological rigor (RCTs vs pretest–posttest trials) of the studies. The author also found the CBT effect sizes of anxiety with Black individuals to be analogous to meta-analysis consisting of person who were primarily White.

Another meta-analysis has examined the effects of third wave CBT, mindfulness and acceptance-based CBT for depressive symptoms with Black individuals (Dawson et al., 2022). As with the previous two CBT meta-analyses for Black individuals (Gregory Jr., 2016, 2019), Dawson and associates' meta-analysis was also limited by the lack of primary studies which included Black individuals. The studies included in the meta-analysis were categorized according to the percentage of Black individuals within each primary study. The meta-analysis included youth and adults. The results showed that mindfulness and acceptance-based CBT interventions were associated with small to medium positive effects in the Black participants. The meta-analysis also showed that the effect of mindfulness and acceptance-based CBT differed significantly by age and geography. Adults had a moderate effect, while youth had a small effect. The biggest effects of mindfulness and acceptance-based CBT were seen in the southeast region of the United States. A number of meta-analyses addressed internalized disorders in youth (Cougle & Grubaugh, 2022; Huey & Polo, 2008), however, given the purpose and/or methods of those meta-analyses, their utility for determining the efficacy of CBT for Black individuals was substantially limited.

1.7.3 Meta-Analyses of Substance Use Disorders

The most prevalent meta-analytic examination of CBT for an externalized disorder, addressed substance use. The CBT meta-analyses addressing substance use disorders with Black individuals yielded positive outcomes overall; however, there were a number of factors that hampered these findings. The meta-analysis by Windsor and associates (2015) provided the most transparent assessment of CBT for substance use among Black individuals. The CBT meta-analysis conducted by Windsor and colleagues examined substance use outcomes and included RCTs. However, it did have several limitations. Black and Hispanic samples were combined, thereby somewhat limiting the generalizability of the results to Black individuals. The meta-analysis found that for Black and Hispanic individuals, CBT demonstrated large, statistically significant reductions in substance use with within-group, pretest–posttest analysis. However, when analyses were based on between-group, CBT versus control comparisons, there was no statistically significant difference, and the effect was substantially small. The meta-analysis also found that Black and Hispanic participants did not significantly differ from non-Hispanic White participants in engagement, retention, or follow-up. A meta-analysis addressing tobacco use in exclusive samples of Black Americans showed a significant reduction in tobacco use (Montgomery et al., 2017); however, some trials that did not use a CBT intervention were included. Meta-analytic examinations of external disorders in Black youth (Cougle & Grubaugh, 2022; Huey & Polo, 2008) had substantially less utility for determining CBT's efficacy in Black individuals because the studies included multiple racial groups and/or multiple interventions.

1.7.4 Meta-Analyses of Culturally Adapted Cognitive-Behavioral Therapy

The initial development and dissemination of CBT was conducted by members of the majority culture who were predominantly White and Protestant (Stone et al., 2018). Yet, over time, Beckian, second-wave CBT has grown to be adapted to address anxious, traumatic, and psychotic issues experienced by different cultural groups (Naeem, 2019). Specific culturally adapted CBTs for Black Americans have focused on diagnostic categories of depression (Neblett et al., 2018) and anxiety (Carter & Sbrocco, 2018). Clinical researchers continue to ask whether CBT should be culturally adapted for Black and other non-White racial groups (Huey Jr et al., 2023)? While some research has suggested that non-adapted CBT may be sufficient for Black individuals (Markell et al., 2014), a larger body of research supports the use of culturally adapted interventions. Several narrative reviews (Huey Jr et al., 2014, 2023) and meta-analyses (Hall et al., 2016) have focused exclusively on culturally adapted psychotherapy and the results have been favorable overall. Although the applicability of this research to Black Americans is somewhat limited. In literature reviews, Huey and colleagues (Huey Jr et al., 2014, 2023) have documented meta-analytic research supporting the efficacy of CBT for non-White racial groups and conducted some of the most comprehensive research on the topic of cultural adaptions in CBT. The 2014 review conducted by Huey and associates found culturally adapted CBT to have overall efficacy. However, the 2014 review by Huey and associates was not limited to Black individuals, thereby decreasing the study's ability to answer the question of does CBT need to be adapted for Black Americans. A meta-analysis conducted by Hall and colleagues (2016) provided a more precise examination via estimating the magnitude of effect for culturally adapted interventions. Yet, as it pertains to the question at hand, this meta-analysis was also limited by its broad inclusion of other races and lack of specificity to Black individuals. In this meta-analysis, CBT was the most frequently used intervention and 29% of the individuals in the meta-analysis were of African descent. The authors of this meta-analysis found that the overall effect was moderate and favored culturally adapted interventions.

A meta-analysis by Silveus and associates (Silveus et al., 2023) specifically examined culturally adapted CBT for depression and anxiety. The meta-analysis found that culturally adapted CBT had moderate, positive effects on depression and anxiety. The meta-analysis showed culturally adapted CBT as having large effects for anxiety and depression reduction. However, this meta-analysis also combined all racial and ethnic groups, therefore limiting specific conclusions that could be drawn for CBT for Black Americans. A culturally adapted therapy meta-analysis in 2006 (Griner & Smith, 2006) showed culturally adapted therapy was moderately beneficial relative unadapted therapy. The meta-analysis by Griner and Smith, examined the effect of culturally adapted psychotherapy on African Americans alone, and the outcomes remained moderate; however, CBT was not required for a study to be included in the meta-analysis. The culturally adapted meta-analysis conducted by Benish et al., (2011) had a small effect that favored the use of culturally adapted therapy for various psychosocial outcomes, relative to traditional psychotherapy. However, this meta-analysis was not necessarily limited to CBT and the meta-analysis combined different racial and ethnic groups, thereby limiting the ability to draw conclusions about culturally adapted CBT for Black Americans. In summary, despite the tentative favorability of these meta-analyses on culturally adapted therapy for various mental health outcomes, there are a number of factors that limit the utility of these findings for Black Americans being treated with CBT. One of the biggest issues in these meta-analyses (Benish et al., 2011; Silveus et al., 2023) was the tendency to analyze different racial and ethnic groups in the same analysis. The results of these culturally adapted CBT meta-analyses would be more useful if subgroup analyses were conducted that looked at the effects of the culturally adapted CBT for each race that was included in the meta-analysis. Therefore, although the meta-analyses have found some positive results for culturally adapted therapy, the specific impact of culturally adapted CBT for Black Americans requires more research.

1.8 The Gap Between Cognitive-Behavioral Research and Black American Mental Health

Despite some positive meta-analytic findings, CBT has been legitimately critiqued on a number of issues related to culture. The aforementioned lack of Black-relevant CBT research is a limitation of CBT for Black Americans, however, not one that precludes its use (Gregory Jr. & Clary, 2022). Cognitive-behavioral therapy's emphasis on science, objectivity, and individualistic values may contrast with the values of some cultures (Beck, 2021). Although it is worth noting the uniqueness of Black American individuals and the value of the within-group diversity of the Black American culture (see Chap. 4 for further discussion). Black Americans have developed a collective identity that has provided a robust response to various forms of oppression (Ogbu, 2004). However, research has shown some evidence of Black Americans having both individualistic and collectivist attributes (Riley-Eddins & Jackson, 1999; Smith et al., 2019). For example, Black children expressed significantly more individualistic values than their White counterparts, and there was no difference in collectivist values between the two racial groups (Smith et al., 2019). Research regarding Black American female coping has shown a variety of coping characteristics that are at times contrary to the collectivist culture (Riley-Eddins & Jackson, 1999). Additionally, there are aspects of a collectivist Black American culture that could be compatible and even synergistic with cognitive interventions. Chapter 6, *Cognitive-Behavioral Interventions with Black Americans*, provides a discussion of the cognitive model and cognitive interventions within a Black American collectivist culture as well as the synergistic impact of behavioral interventions. As previously mentioned, there is evidence to suggest that the implementation of cognitive restructuring by therapists with Black individuals could be viewed as less important or underused (Ezawa & Strunk, 2022a, 2022b). The clinician's own cultural biases are also factors that can negatively impact CBT with Black Americans (Beck, 2021). Some of these issues, which may negatively impact therapeutic work with Black Americans will be addressed in Chap. 3 (*Cognitive-Behavioral Therapy and Implicit Racial Bias*) and Chap. 4 (*Cognitive-Behavioral Principles for Black Americans*), in a subsection titled "Traditional Cognitive-Behavioral Principles: Congruence with Black American Issues."

1.9 Cognitive-Behavioral Therapy for Black Americans: Gaps in Treatment Literature

Cognitive-behavioral texts, solely devoted to CBT with Black Americans, would be crucial in addressing Black American traumas, mental health disparities, and the implications of structural racism. A number of edited books (Chang et al., 2018; Iwamasa & Hays, 2019; Jones, 2004; Wells-Wilbon & Estreet, 2022) and sole-authored books (Beck, 2016) have made meaningful contributions to issues of psychotherapy and race. However, the lack of intervention or racial exclusivity on CBT and Black Americans, respectively, may make their utility to Black Americans being treated with CBT less applicable. An edited book by Turner and Jones (1982), *Behavior Modification in Black Populations: Psychosocial Issues and Empirical Findings*, has a strong behavioral emphasis and therefore focuses more on the first wave of CBT. However, the edited text did include one chapter on rational emotive behavioral therapy (Maultsby Jr., 1982). *Anxiety disorders in African Americans* (Friedman, 1994) included coverage of CBT for specific anxiety diagnoses. DeLapp (2025) has a self-help book that addresses racial and cultural stress. Another recent text by Steele (2025), discusses CBT with Black Americans and centers on racism. However, the structural context of racism and its specific implications for CBT providers and Black clients remain a necessary and valuable contribution to the therapeutic literature.

1.10 Cognitive-Behavioral Therapy with Black Americans: A Principle and Structurally Informed Perspective—Purpose and Structure of the Book

The author of the book has years of experience using CBT and working with Black Americans in various clinical environments, primarily outpatient therapeutic settings. The author has previously described the lack of clinically relevant research and professional literature that is available to benefit clinicians who are working with Black Americans (Gregory Jr. & Tucker Edmonds, 2023). When providing clinical services, the author had experiences with Black American clients, colleagues, and administration that suggested a need to discuss cognitive-behavioral therapy in the context of structural racism. Although cognitive-behavioral research for Black Americans is limited, research has been conducted to generate thematic patterns for improving practice with Black Americans in CBT. Clinicians may very well benefit from a framework that provides an integration of research findings pertinent to CBT for Black Americans. As a university professor, the author has seen the need to develop clinically relevant resources for graduate students who may very well work with Black Americans, using CBT, in different clinical settings. The needs of graduate students working with Black Americans include but are not limited to: understanding the extant clinical research regarding Black American clients, therapeutic engagement with Black American clients, the students' own beliefs about Black clients and Black culture, culturally relevant assessment tools, creating cognitive-behavioral case conceptualizations, and applying cognitive-behavioral interventions with Black American clients. Similar to clinicians, graduate students in the helping professions can also benefit greatly from a framework that embodies the most important components of CBT with Black American clients. As a clinical researcher, the author's studies examine CBT with Black Americans using a number of methods: systematic reviews, meta-analyses, qualitative research, psychometrics, and statistical modeling. A text that provides a summary of cognitive-behavioral research for Black Americans across a number of methodologies and a text that provides a unifying framework for cognitive-behavioral principles for Black Americans has several uses. The present text could be used as a basis to identify and explore different research questions that ultimately advance the external validity of CBT findings for Black Americans.

The purpose of the book is to provide principles for tailoring CBT to Black Americans experiencing psychiatric and/or QOL issues while acknowledging and addressing the impact of structural racism. The present text seeks to comprehensively address principles, empirical, and application issues of CBT for Black Americans within the context of structural racism. The term "Black Americans" must be operationally defined. Although race is often thought of as biological in nature, race is a social construct (Bryant et al., 2022). Black Americans are defined as individuals within the US who have ancestry in the Black African racial groups (US Census Bureau, 2022). Therefore, Black Americans also include Black Hispanics and multiracial individuals with Black ancestors. The term "Black Americans" is used in the title and throughout the book; however with few exceptions, the overall principles and applications should be transferable to other nations with Black individuals who experience the simultaneous tension among structural forces and the implementation of CBT. The final chapter of the text discusses how the cognitive behavioral principles may be relevant for other Black diasporic groups.

Principle-informed CBT with Black American is needed to aid in harmonizing structural inequity, diverse and resilient Black cultural attributes, and clinicians' desire to effectively use CBT with Black Americans. A principle-informed CBT approach has the advantages of efficiently addressing diagnostic comorbidity (Newman, 2020) and multilevel psychosocial influences, which may threaten therapeutic rapport or complicate the implementation of CBT interventions with Black Americans. The principles are methodically developed, empirically based, practical tools that may be used to aid clinical decision-making. The principles should not replace legal, ethical, or otherwise sound-clinical judgment and supervision. Throughout the book, research and applications are provided to enhance practical implementation of the CBT principles for Black Americans. The book is divided into three sections. The chapters in the subsequent sections make substantive use of research, principles, and application to achieve the overall purpose of the book. Part I of the book addresses the historical and present, context of CBT with African Americans (Chaps. 1 and 2). Part II addresses implicit racial bias, CBT principles for Black Americans, and the CBT principles' manifestations in cognitive and behavioral interventions (Chaps. 3, 4, 5, 6 and 7). Part III provides applications for Black men, women, and diasporic groups (Chap. 8).

The present chapter has summarized the compelling progress and success of CBT, which has been documented across a number of disorders (Butler et al., 2006; David et al., 2018; Hofmann et al., 2012). Over the last two decades there has been incremental systematic review and meta-analytic research evidence that collectively provides some support for CBT's potential to efficaciously address psychosocial issues among Black individuals (Dawson et al., 2022; Gregory Jr., 2016, 2019; Horrell, 2008; Montgomery et al., 2017; Windsor et al., 2015). Yet, Black individuals overall, have not fully realized the potential psychiatric and QOL benefits which CBT may offer. With this disparity in mind, this chapter has also provided an overview of stakeholders and Black gaps in treatment and research, which may benefit from cognitive-behavioral principles which target Black Americans addressing psychiatric and QOL issues in the context of structural racism. In the broader context of social–environmental issues, the American Psychological Association (APA) has provided guidelines addressing psychologists' roles in race and ethnicity (APA, 2017, 2019). These guidelines are substantive, yet they lack interdisciplinary relevance, and they are not specific to CBT and the unique issues experienced by Black individuals. To address the lack of CBT principles or guidelines for Black individuals with psychiatric and QOL issues, the subsequent chapters of this book fill this gap in cognitive-behavioral literature.

Chapter 2 provides an overview of structural and systemic factors that create Black trauma and sustain Black intrapersonal and interpersonal suffering. Specific Black manifestations of anxiety, depression, and opioid use are linked to structural and systemic catalysts. For Black clients, cognitive-behavioral interventions occur within the context of anti-Black structural racism. Cognitive-behavioral therapy has the potential to empower Black clients and foster resilience that counters the negative synergy that exists between psychiatric morbidity and anti-Black structural racism. The second chapter summarizes expectations for what can be accomplished using CBT with Black clients in an anti-Black or colorblind (Bonilla-Silva & Forman, 2000) ecosystem.

Chapter 3 examines the role of implicit racial bias in cognitive-behavioral clinicians. The ways in which implicit racial bias may manifest itself are described and multilevel methods for reducing implicit racial bias in cognitive-behavioral clinicians are discussed. Chapter 3's focus on implicit racial bias is viewed as a necessary prerequisite to the discussion of cognitive-behavioral principles for Black Americans. By first addressing implicit racial bias, the reader will be primed for the presentation of cognitive-behavioral principles for Black Americans.

Chapter 4 introduces ten Black-specific cognitive-behavioral principles that are used to guide CBT with Black individuals addressing psychiatric and/or QOL issues in the context of structural racism. These Black-specific, cognitive-behavioral principles are congruent with and used to support and enhance foundational principles which have already been articulated in CBT (Beck, 2021). The cognitive-behavioral Black principles are collectively represented by the mnemonic acronym, RESPPECTUS (see Table 4.1 in Chap. 4 and Appendix B) and address factors of therapeutic rapport and cognitive-behavioral intervention with Black individuals addressing mental health or QOL issues in the context of structural racism. The principles represent the basic guidelines for CBT with Black Americans.

The purpose of Chap. 5 is to aid clinicians in efficiently selecting and using psychometrically appropriate scales for practice and research, as well as to develop cognitive-behavioral case conceptualizations for Black American Clients. Cognitive-behavioral therapy has an emphasis on interventions which target latent variables (thoughts, beliefs; Naragon-Gainey & Brown, 2015). When scales that have not been previously validated with Black samples are used to measure latent variables in Black individuals, there is a potential for the scale's measurement properties to vary according to race or other cultural factors (Bryne, 2016). Therefore, the psychometric properties of scales which have been validated in Black samples are provided in a tabular and narrative format. Readers will need to identify and abide by the intellectual property rights of each of the identified scales in Chap. 4. Additionally, in this chapter the Cultural Trauma Scale (CuTS; Gregory Jr. & Tucker Edmonds, 2024a, 2024b), is discussed and its two versions are provided in Appendices C and D. In Chap. 5, a hypothetical vignette is provided that is loosely based on the author's years of experience with working with Black clients using CBT in various settings. This vignette was used to demonstrate how the CuTS and other measures could be used in cognitive-behavioral case conceptualization for Black clients.

In Chap. 6, cognitive factors which mediate structural forces and undesirable emotions are identified and defined. Chapter 6 discusses the cognitive model within the context of Black American cultural factors and cognitive restructuring interventions based on the framework of the RESPPECTUS Principles. Behavioral interventions with Black individuals, based on the RESPPECTUS principles, are explicated. Within Chap. 6, the hypothetical vignette that was discussed in Chap. 5 is used to illustrate the application of the RESPPECTUS principles with cognitive and behavioral interventions for a Black male young adult client.

Chapter 7 discusses the use of the RESPPECTUS principles in the context of cognitive-behavioral group therapy with Black Americans. The relationship between CBT, Yalom's Therapeutic Factors (Yalom & Leszcz, 2020), and Black Americans is discussed. The cognitive-behavioral RESPPECTUS principles for Black Americans in group therapy are also delineated. The last chapter is used to address intersectional applications of CBT with Black individuals. Chapter 8 provides specific intersectional disparities, methods for improving engagement, and cognitive-behavioral approaches for Black men and women. Chapter 8 also examines the extent to which the ten RESPPECTUS principles could be used with other individuals throughout the Black diaspora. While basic knowledge in cognitive-behavioral theory and practice is helpful, the book does not assume that readers have a prerequisite CBT knowledge base. Therefore, fundamental aspects of CBT are explained, and readers are provided with references should they wish to acquire additional knowledge on the foundational topics. The book is intended to be used with graduate students and mental health professionals (with appropriate licensure and supervision) belonging to various professional disciplines and subgroups: clinical social work, clinical and social psychology, psychiatry, counseling, marriage and family therapy, nursing, public health, and others. Researchers addressing clinically oriented questions regarding Black individuals, families, and/or communities will also find the content of the book vital for their work.

1.11 The Historical Context of Cognitive-Behavioral Therapy with Black Americans: Summary

By reviewing a brief history of CBT with Black Americans, the foundation is provided for further discussion in the proceeding chapters. While under-researched, the extant systematic review and meta-analytic research demonstrate CBT has promise for Black Americans experiencing various mental health, substance use issues, and racial stressors. This chapter includes brief discussions of CBT from the perspectives of the clinicians and Black clients. Finally, an overview of the organization of the book was provided. Appendix A provides readers with a list of empirical articles and reviews regarding CBT with Black Americans. The next chapter examines CBT in the context of anti-Black structural racism within the United States. Cognitive-behavioral therapy with Black Americans occurs within the context of historical and contemporary structures, institutions, laws, policies, and intersecting cultures. Chapter 2 uses an ecological systems theory (Bronfenbrenner, 1977) to provide a framework for explaining the mechanisms by which anti-Black structural racism impacts the lives of Black Americans and ultimately the CBT process.

References

Allen, J. D., Shelton, R. C., Emmons, K. M., & Linnan, L. A. (2018). Fidelity and its relationship to effectiveness, adaptation, and dissemination. In R. C. Brownson, G. A. Colditz, & E. K. Proctor (Eds.), *Dissemination and implementation in research in health: Translating science to practice* (2nd ed., pp. 267–284). Oxford University Press.

American Psychological Association. 2017. Multicultural guidelines: An ecological approach to context, identity, and intersectionality. Retrieved from: http://www.apa.org/about/policy/multicultural-guidelines.pdf

American Psychological Association, APA Task Force on Race and Ethnicity Guidelines in Psychology. (2019). *Race and ethnicity guidelines in psychology: Promoting responsiveness and equity*. Retrieved from https://www.apa.org/about/policy/guidelines-race-ethnicity.pdf

Beck, A. (2016). *Transcultural cognitive behaviour therapy for anxiety and depression: A practical guide*. Routledge.

Beck, A. T. (1952). Successful outpatient psychotherapy of a chronic schizophrenic with a delusion based on borrowed guilt. *Psychiatry, 15*, 305–312.

Beck, A. T. (1976). *Cognitive therapy and the emotional disorders*. Meridian.

Beck, A. T., Davis, D. D., & Freeman, A. (Eds.). (2015). *Cognitive therapy of personality disorders* (3rd ed.). Guilford Press.

Beck, A. T., Emery, G., & Greenberg, R. L. (1985). *Anxiety disorders and phobias: A cognitive perspective*. Basic Books.

Beck, A. T., Rector, N. A., Stolar, N., & Grant, P. (2009). *Schizophrenia: Cognitive theory, research, and therapy*. Guilford Press.

Beck, A. T., Rush, A. J., Shaw, B. F., & Emery, G. (1979). *Cognitive therapy of depression*. Guilford Press.

Beck, A. T., Wright, F. D., Newman, C. F., & Liese, B. S. (1993). *Cognitive therapy of substance abuse*. Guilford Press.

Beck, J. S. (2021). *Cognitive behavior therapy: Basics and beyond* (3rd ed.). Guilford Press.

Benish, S. G., Quintana, S., & Wampold, B. E. (2011). Culturally adapted psychotherapy and the legitimacy of myth: A direct-comparison meta-analysis. *Journal of Counseling Psychology, 58*(3), 279–289.

Bonilla-Silva, E., & Forman, T. A. (2000). "I am not a racist but…": Mapping White college students' racial ideology in the USA. *Discourse & Society, 11*(1), 50–85. https://doi.org/10.1177/0957926500011001003

Borenstein, M., Hedges, L. V., Higgins, J. P. T., & Rothstein, H. R. (2021). *Introduction to meta-analysis* (2nd ed.). John Wiley & Sons.

Bronfenbrenner, U. (1977). Toward an experimental ecology of human development. *American Psychologist, 32*(7), 513–531. https://doi.org/10.1037/0003-066X.32.7.513

Bryant, B. E., Jordan, A., & Clark, U. S. (2022). Race as a social construct in psychiatry research and practice. *JAMA Psychiatry, 79*(2), 93–94. https://doi.org/10.1001/jamapsychiatry.2021.2877

Bryne, B. M. (2016). *Structural equation modeling with Amos: Basic concepts, applications, and programming* (3rd ed.). Taylor & Francis.

Butler, A. C., Chapman, J. E., Forman, E. M., & Beck, A. T. (2006). The empirical status of cognitive-behavioral therapy: A review of meta-analyses. *Clinical Psychology Review, 26*(1), 17–31. https://doi.org/10.1016/j.cpr.2005.07.003

Carter, M. M., & Sbrocco, T. (2018). Cognitive behavioral models, measures, and treatments for anxiety disorders in African Americans. In E. C. Chang, C. A. Downey, J. K. Hirsch, & E. A. Yu (Eds.), *Treating depression, anxiety, and stress in ethnic and racial groups: Cognitive behavioral approaches* (pp. 179–202). American Psychological Association. https://doi.org/10.1037/0000091-008

Cather, C., Penn, D., Otto, M., & Goff, D. C. (2004). Cognitive therapy for delusions in schizophrenia: Models, benefits, and new approaches. *Journal of Cognitive Psychotherapy, 18*(3), 207–221. https://doi.org/10.1891/jcop.18.3.207.65650

Chang, E. C., Downey, C. A., Kirsch, J. K., & Yu, E. A. (2018). *Treating depression, anxiety, and stress in ethnic and racial groups: Cognitive behavioral approaches*. American Psychological Association.

Cougle, J. R., & Grubaugh, A. L. (2022). Do psychosocial treatment outcomes vary by race or ethnicity? A review of meta-analyses. *Clinical Psychology Review, 96*, 1–8. https://doi.org/10.1016/j.cpr.2022.102192

David, D., Cristea, I., & Hofmann, S. G. (2018). Why cognitive Behavioral therapy is the current gold standard of psychotherapy. *Frontiers in Psychiatry, 9*, 4. https://doi.org/10.3389/fpsyt.2018.00004

Dawson, D. N., Jones, M. C., Fairbairn, C. E., & Laurent, H. K. (2022). Mindfulness and acceptance-based interventions with Black Americans: A meta-analysis of intervention efficacy for depressive symptoms. *Journal of Consulting and Clinical Psychology, 90*(2), 123–136. https://doi.org/10.1037/ccp0000706.supp

DeLapp, R. C. T. (2025). *Empower yourself against racial and cultural stress using skills from the REACH program to cope, heal, and thrive*. Guilford Press.

Edge, D., & Lemetyinen, H. (2019). Psychology across cultures: Challenges and opportunities. *Psychology & Psychotherapy: Theory, Research & Practice, 92*(2), 261–276. https://doi.org/10.1111/papt.12229

Ellis, A. (1994). *Reason and emotion in psychotherapy: A comprehensive method of treating human disturbances (revised and updated)*. Carol Publishing Group.

Ezawa, I. D., & Strunk, D. R. (2022a). Working with Black vs. white patients: An experimental test of therapist decision-making in cognitive behavioral therapy for depression. *Cognitive Behaviour Therapy, 51*(3), 229–242. https://doi.org/10.1080/16506073.2021.1970799

Ezawa, I. D., & Strunk, D. R. (2022b). Differences in the delivery of cognitive Behavioral therapy for depression when therapists work with Black and White patients. *Cognitive Therapy & Research, 46*(1), 104–113. https://doi.org/10.1007/s10608-021-10254-0

Fairburn, C. G. (2008). *Cognitive behavior therapy and eating disorders*. Guilford Press.

Fordham, B., Sugavanam, T., Edwards, K., Stallard, P., Howard, R., das Nair, R., Copsey, B., Lee, H., Howick, J., Hemming, K., & Lamb, S. E. (2021). The evidence for cognitive behavioural therapy in any condition, population or context: A meta-review of systematic reviews and panoramic meta-analysis. *Psychological Medicine, 51*(1), 21–29. https://doi.org/10.1017/S0033291720005292

Free, M. L. (1999). *Cognitive therapy in groups: Guidelines and resources for practice*. John Wiley & Sons.

Friedman, S. (Ed.). (1994). *Anxiety disorders in African Americans*. Springer Publishing Company.

Gambrill, E. D. (1994). Concepts and methods of behavioral treatment. In D. K. Granvold (Ed.), *Cognitive and behavioral treatment: Methods and applications* (pp. 32–62). Wadsworth.

Glass, G. V. (1976). Primary, secondary, and meta-analysis of research. *Educational Researcher, 5*(10), 3–8.

Granvold, D. K. (1994). Concepts and methods of cognitive treatment. In D. K. Granvold (Ed.), *Cognitive and behavioral treatment: Methods and applications* (pp. 3–31). Wadsworth.

Gregory, V. L., Jr. (2016). Cognitive-behavioral therapy for depressive symptoms in persons of African descent: A meta-analysis. *Journal of Social Service Research, 42*(1), 113–129. https://doi.org/10.1080/01488376.2015.1084973

Gregory, V. L., Jr. (2019). Cognitive-behavioral therapy for anxious symptoms in persons of African descent: A meta-analysis. *Journal of Social Service Research, 45*(1), 87–101. https://doi.org/10.1080/01488376.2018.1479344

Gregory, V. L. (2021).Cognitive-behavioral therapy for relationship distress: Meta-analysis of RCTs with social work implications. *Journal of Evidence-Based Social Work, 18*(1), 49–70. https://doi.org/10.1080/26408066.2020.1806164

Gregory, V. L., Jr., & Clary, K. L. (2022). Addressing anti-Black racism: The roles of social work. *Smith College Studies In Social Work, 92*(1), 1–27. https://doi.org/10.1080/00377317.2021.2008287

Gregory, V. L., Jr., & Tucker Edmonds, J. L. (2023). The racial pandemic experienced by Black American men: Cognitive-behavioral and structural implications. *American Journal of Orthopsychiatry, 93*(1), 1–16. https://doi.org/10.1037/ort0000651

Gregory, V. L., Jr., & Tucker Edmonds, J. L. (2024a). Cultural trauma scale: Psychometric evaluation of Black men's beliefs, emotions, and coping. *Psychological Trauma: Theory, Research, Practice, and Policy, 16*(8), 1329–1337. https://doi.org/10.1037/tra0001607

Gregory, V. L., Jr., & Tucker Edmonds, J. L. (2024b). Cultural trauma scale (CuTS): Parsimonious principal component analysis, independent Black American male sample. *Journal of Aggression, Maltreatment & Trauma, 33*(3), 369–386. https://doi.org/10.1080/10926771.2023.2256741

Griner, D., & Smith, T. B. (2006). Culturally adapted mental health intervention: A meta-analytic review. *Psychotherapy: Theory, Research, Practice, Training, 43*(4), 531–548. https://doi.org/10.1037/0033-3204.43.4.531

Gurpinar-Morgan, A., Murray, C., & Beck, A. (2014). Ethnicity and the therapeutic relationship: Views of young people accessing cognitive behavioural therapy. *Mental Health, Religion & Culture, 17*(7), 714–725. https://doi.org/10.1080/13674676.2014.903388

Hall, G. C. N., Ibaraki, A. Y., Huang, E. R., Marti, C. N., & Stice, E. (2016). A meta-analysis of cultural adaptations of psychological interventions. *Behavior Therapy, 47*(6), 993–1014. https://doi.org/10.1016/j.beth.2016.09.005

Hayes, S. C. (2016). Acceptance and commitment therapy, relational frame theory, and the third wave of Behavioral and cognitive therapies–republished article. *Behavior Therapy, 47*(6), 869–885. https://doi.org/10.1016/j.beth.2016.11.006

Hayes, S. C., Strosahl, K. D., & Wilson, K. G. (2012). *Acceptance and commitment therapy: The process of practice and mindful change* (2nd ed.). Guilford Press.

Hofmann, S. G., Asnaani, A., Vonk, I. J. J., Sawyer, A. T., & Fang, A. (2012). The efficacy of cognitive behavioral therapy: A review of meta-analyses. *Cognitive Therapy and Research, 36*(5), 427–440. https://doi.org/10.1007/s10608-012-9476-1

Horrell, S. C. V. (2008). Effectiveness of cognitive-behavioral therapy with adult ethnic minority clients: A review. *Professional Psychology: Research and Practice, 39*(2), 160–168. https://doi.org/10.1037/0735-7028.39.2.160

Huey, S. J., Jr., Park, A. L., Galán, C. A., & Wang, C. X. (2023). Culturally responsive cognitive Behavioral therapy for ethnically diverse populations. *Annual Review of Clinical Psychology, 19*, 51–78. https://doi.org/10.1146/annurev-clinpsy-080921-072750

Huey, S. J., Jr., Tilley, J. L., Jones, E. O., & Smith, C. A. (2014). The contribution of cultural competence to evidence-based care for ethnically diverse populations. *Annual Review of Clinical Psychology, 10*, 305–338. https://doi.org/10.1146/annurev-clinpsy-032813-153729

Huey, S., & Polo, A. (2008). Evidence-based psychosocial treatments for ethnic minority youth. *Journal of Clinical Child & Adolescent Psychology, 37*(1), 262–301. https://doi.org/10.1080/15374410701820174

Ishikawa, S. (2015). A cognitive-behavioral model of anxiety disorders in children and adolescents. *Japanese Psychological Research, 57*(3), 180–193. https://doi.org/10.1111/jpr.12078

Iwamasa, G. Y., & Hays, P. A. (Eds.). (2019). *Culturally responsive cognitive-behavioral therapy* (2nd ed.). American Psychological Association.

Johnsen, T. J., & Thimm, J. C. (2018). A meta-analysis of group cognitive-Behavioral therapy as an Antidepressive treatment: Are we getting better? *Canadian Psychology, 59*(1), 15–30. https://doi.org/10.1037/cap0000132

Jones, R. (Ed.). (2004). *Black psychology* (4th ed.). Cobb & Henry.

Koffel, E. A., Koffel, J. B., & Gehrman, P. R. (2015). A meta-analysis of group cognitive behavioral therapy for insomnia. *Sleep Medicine Reviews, 19*, 6–16. https://doi.org/10.1016/j.smrv.2014.05.001

Lampard, A. M., Tasca, G. A., Balfour, L., & Bissada, H. (2013). An evaluation of the Transdiagnostic cognitive-behavioural model of eating disorders. *European Eating Disorders Review, 21*(2), 99–107. https://doi.org/10.1002/erv.2214

Leahy, R. (1996). *Cognitive therapy: Basic principles and applications*. Jason Aronson.

Linehan, M. M. (1993). *Cognitive-behavioral treatment of borderline personality disorder*. Guilford Press.

Markell, H. M., Newman, M. G., Gallop, R., Gibbons, M. B., Rickels, K., & Crits-Christoph, P. (2014). Combined medication and CBT for generalized anxiety disorder with African American participants: Reliability and validity of assessments and preliminary outcomes. *Behavior Therapy, 45*(4), 495–506. https://doi.org/10.1016/j.beth.2014.02.008

Maultsby, M. C., Jr. (1982). Rational behavior therapy. In S. M. Turner & R. T. Jones (Eds.), *Behavior modification in Black populations: Psychosocial issues and empirical findings* (pp. 151–170). Springer.

McMain, S., Newman, M. G., Segal, Z. V., & DeRubeis, R. J. (2015). Cognitive behavioral therapy: Current status and future research directions. *Psychotherapy Research, 25*(3), 321–329. https://doi.org/10.1080/10503307.2014.1002440

Meichenbaum, D. (1977). *Cognitive-behavior modification*. Plenum Press. https://doi.org/10.1007/978-1-4757-9739-8

Montgomery, L., Robinson, C., Seaman, E. L., & Haeny, A. M. (2017). A scoping review and meta-analysis of psychosocial and pharmacological treatments for cannabis and tobacco use among African Americans. *Psychology of Addictive Behaviors, 31*(8), 922–943. https://doi.org/10.1037/adb0000326

Naeem, F. (2019). Cultural adaptations of CBT: A summary and discussion of the special issue on cultural adaptation of CBT. *Cognitive Behaviour Therapist, 12*, 1–20. https://doi.org/10.1017/S1754470X19000278

Naragon-Gainey, K., & Brown, T. A. (2015). Enhancing measurement validation in cognitive clinical research with structural equation modeling and item response theory. In G. P. Brown & D. A. Clark (Eds.), *Assessment in cognitive therapy* (pp. 268–290). Guilford Press.

Neblett, E. W., Sosoo, E. E., Willis, H. A., Bernard, D. L., Bae, J., Chang, E. C., Downey, C. A., Hirsch, J. K., & Yu, E. A. (2018). Treating depression anxiety and stress in ethnic and racial groups: Cognitive behavioral approaches. Cognitive behavioral models measures and treatments for depressive disorders in African Americans. *American Psychological Association Washington*, 73–97.

Newman, C. F. (2020). Principle-informed CBT in a complex case. *Cognitive and Behavioral Practice, 27*(4), 360–376. https://doi.org/10.1016/j.cbpra.2020.04.001

Nichols, M. P., & Davis, S. D. (2017). *Family therapy: Concepts and methods* (11th ed.). Pearson.

Norton, P. J. (2012). *Group cognitive-behavioral therapy of anxiety: A transdiagnostic treatment manual*. Guilford Press.

Norton, P. J., & Paulus, D. J. (2017). Transdiagnostic models of anxiety disorder: Theoretical and empirical underpinnings. *Clinical Psychology Review, 56*, 122–137. https://doi.org/10.1016/j.cpr.2017.03.004

Ogbu, J. U. (2004). Collective identity and the burden of "acting white" in Black history, community, and education. *Urban Review, 36*(1), 1–35. https://doi.org/10.1023/B:URRE.0000042734.83194.f6

Olfson, M., Zuvekas, S. H., McClellan, C., Wall, M. M., Hankerson, S. H., & Blanco, C. (2023). Racial-ethnic disparities in outpatient mental health Care in the United States. *Psychiatric Services (Washington, D.C.), 74*(7), 674. https://doi.org/10.1176/appi.ps.20220365

Overholser, J. C. (2010). Psychotherapy according to the Socratic method: Integrating ancient philosophy with contemporary cognitive therapy. *Journal of Cognitive Psychotherapy, 24*(4), 354–363. https://doi.org/10.1891/0889-8391.24.4.354

Padgett, D. K. (2017). *Qualitative methods in social work research: Challenges and rewards*. Sage Publications.

Pössel, P., & Black, S. W. (2014). Testing three different sequential mediational interpretations of Beck's cognitive model of the development of depression. *Journal of Clinical Psychology, 70*(1), 72–94. https://doi.org/10.1002/jclp.22001

Rathod, S., Kingdon, D., Phiri, P., & Gobbi, M. (2010). Developing culturally sensitive cognitive behaviour therapy for psychosis for ethnic minority patients by exploration and incorporation of service users' and health professionals' views and opinions. *Behavioural and Cognitive Psychotherapy, 38*(5), 511–533. https://doi.org/10.1017/S1352465810000378

Rathus, J. H., & Sanderson, W. C. (1999). *Marital distress: Cognitive behavioral interventions for couples*. Jason Aronson.

Raylu, N., Oei, T. P. S., Loo, J. M. Y., & Tsai, J.-S. (2016). Testing the validity of a cognitive behavioral model for gambling behavior. *Journal of Gambling Studies, 32*(2), 773–788. https://doi.org/10.1007/s10899-015-9567-5

Riley-Eddins, E. A., & Jackson, A. (1999). Ethnicity and coping: The multiaxial model of coping. *Journal of Multicultural Nursing & Health (JMCNH), 5*(1), 27–35.

Sank, L. I., & Shaffer, C. S. (1984). *A therapist's manual for cognitive behavior therapy in groups*. Plenum Press.

Segal, Z., Williams, M., & Teasdale, J. (2013). *Mindfulness-based cognitive therapy for depression* (2nd ed.). Guilford Press.

Silveus, S. A., Schmit, M. K., Oliveira, J. T., & Hughes, L. E. (2023). Meta-analysis of culturally adapted cognitive behavioral therapy for anxiety and depression. *Journal of Counseling & Development, 101*(2), 129–142. https://doi.org/10.1002/jcad.12463

Smith, E. P., Witherspoon, D. P., Bhargava, S., & Bermudez, J. M. (2019). Cultural values and behavior among African American and European American children. *Journal of Child and Family Studies, 28*(5), 1236–1249. https://doi.org/10.1007/s10826-019-01367-y

Steele, J. M. (2025). *Racism and African American mental health: Using cognitive behavior therapy to empower healing*. Routledge.

Stone, L., Beck, A., Hashempour, F., & Thwaites, R. (2018). Introduction to the special issue on cultural adaptations of CBT. *Cognitive Behaviour Therapist, 11*, 1–3. https://doi.org/10.1017/S1754470X18000181

Turner, S. M., & Jones, R. T. (Eds.). (1982). *Behavior modification in Black populations: Psychosocial issues and empirical findings*. Springer.

United States Census Bureau. (2022, March 1). About the topic of race. Retrieved from: https://www.census.gov/topics/population/race/about.html#:~:text=Black%20or%20African%20American%20%E2%80%93%20A,tribal%20affiliation%20or%20community%20attachment

Wells-Wilbon, R., & Estreet, A. (Eds.). (2022). *Trauma and mental health social work with urban populations: African-centered clinical interventions*. Routledge.

Wenzel, A., Liese, B. S., Beck, A. T., & Friedman-Wheeler, D. G. (2012). *Group cognitive therapy for addictions*. The Guilford Press.

Wilson, C. J., & Cottone, R. R. (2013). Using cognitive behavior therapy in clinical work with African American children and adolescents: A review of the literature. *Journal of Multicultural Counseling & Development, 41*(3), 130–143. https://doi.org/10.1002/j.2161-1912.2013.00032.x

Windsor, L. C., Jemal, A., & Alessi, E. J. (2015). Cognitive behavioral therapy: A meta-analysis of race and substance use outcomes. *Cultural Diversity and Ethnic Minority Psychology, 21*(2), 300–313. https://doi.org/10.1037/a0037929

Yalom, I. D., & Leszcz, M. (2020). *The theory and practice of group psychotherapy* (6th ed.). Basic Books/Hachette Book Group.

Young, J. E., Klosko, J. S., & Weishaar, M. E. (2003). *Schema therapy: A practitioner's guide*. The Guilford Press.

Chapter 2
The Structural Context of Cognitive-Behavioral Therapy with Black Americans

2.1 American Anti-Black Structural Racism

Anti-Black racism and various forms of anti-Black discrimination are rooted and have evolved in the United States (Gregory Jr. & Clary, 2022). Throughout American history, the US Constitution (US Senate, n.d.), Black codes, Jim Crow laws, and the criminal justice system embody the prime structures by which Black psychosocial disparities and various forms of Black trauma are created. Beyond the presence of structures which disenfranchise Black Americans directly or indirectly, the disparate implementation of said structures is arguably the biggest contributor to Black disparities and Black distrust of systems. Before discussing the links between structural racism and contemporary Black disparities and negative psychosocial consequences, it is consistent with the principles (Chap. 4) and overall ethos of the book to discuss the rich African heritage from which Black Americans derived.

2.1.1 African Intellectual Contributions Before the Transatlantic Slave Trade

Anthropological research has demonstrated that humanity can trace its origins to the continent of Africa (Gibbons, 2017). However, discussions of Black Americans, in the context of US history, often omit the cultural and intellectual contributions of Black Americans' African origins. These omissions neglect the descendant strengths and contributions to civilization that Black Africans have made prior to the Transatlantic slave trade. Before the Transatlantic slave trade (sixteenth–nineteenth centuries), ancient Africans in Ethiopia created linguistic, governmental, religious, and other scientific knowledge and processes (Jackson, 2017). The intellectual or

V. L. Gregory, Jr., *Cognitive-Behavioral Therapy with Black Americans*,
https://doi.org/10.1007/978-3-032-01666-9_2

scientific contributions include advances in mathematics, astronomy, medicine, architecture, metallurgy, agriculture, and other achievements. With the varied intellectual contributions of Africa, it is not surprising that the first libraries and librarians were established in ancient Egypt ("The Ancient Kemetic Roots of Library and Information Science," 2018). The transatlantic slave trade served as an impediment to African intellectual and technical progress, created in-fighting associated with the enslavement of fellow Africans, and included fiscal and political entropy that laid the foundation for later European colonization (M'baye, 2006). Of the 12.5 million African individuals who were forced into the transatlantic slave trade, 305,326 were brought to the United States (Slave Voyages, 2021).

2.1.2 The United States Constitution: Overt Black American Legal Disenfranchisement

As previously alluded to, there were various structural mechanisms by which enslaved Africans and their descendants were denied freedom, rights, due process, and subjected to various forms of violence and domestic terrorism (Alexander, 2010). The US Constitution never mentions the word "*slavery*," yet there were clear and profound implications for the lives of Black Americans, both enslaved and later free. The United States was conflicted geographically and ideologically, regarding if slavery should be permitted to continue and conflicted by the representation and tax implications of enslaved Africans (Hall & Feldmeier, 2017). It was believed that Whites in the South would find being considered equal with enslaved persons intolerable. This conflict led to a constitutional compromise, where three-fifths of enslaved African persons were counted for taxes and state representation. Ultimately, in addition to being enslaved, embedded in the three-fifths compromise was the inherent, structural dehumanization of Black individuals in America.

2.1.3 The United States Constitution: Circuitous Routes to Black American Legal Disenfranchisement

Beyond the overt denial of dignity and freedom for Black Americans that was embedded in the US Constitution, structural racism and discrimination against Black Americans came in other forms. When the post-US Civil War Reconstruction began, southern states passed Black Codes (Hoag, 2020) and Jim Crow laws (Beermann, 2020) that restricted the rights of Black Americans and resembled some of the legal and humanitarian conditions of slavery. These state-level anti-Black laws were implemented to varying degrees of transparency, thereby varying along a continuum of latent to manifest. In addition to state-based statutes (Black Codes, Jim Crow laws; Beermann, 2020; Hoag, 2020; Koester, 2021), other less conspicuous structures that weakened Constitutional rights for Black Americans came in the forms of case law (Hasbrouck, 2021) and Supreme Court rulings (Beermann, 2020). In the case of state-based statues, these laws provided a legal mechanism for Black Americans to be discriminated against. State-based laws also removed or otherwise limited constitutionally supported rights such as voting or serving on juries for persons who have been convicted of certain crimes (Alexander, 2010; Koester, 2021). Alexander has referred to this mass incarceration dependent, legally sanctioned denial of Black American rights as the *New Jim Crow*. Throughout American history, the large-scale violations of Black Americans' constitutional rights are often most conspicuous in the context of what may be considered various "social problems" (War on Drugs; Alexander, 2010), social movements (Black Lives Matter; Kagan, 2018), or monumental national changes (US Civil War). For example, circuitous violations of Black Americans' 1st (freedom of speech; Kagan, 2018), 4th (protection against unlawful search and seizure; Hasbrouck, 2021), 6th (speedy, public trial and impartial jury; Koester, 2021), 8th (excessive bail, cruel, and unusual punishment; Miller, 2020), 13th amendment (slavery being illegal except for the purpose of punishment for a crime; O'Leary, 2021), 14th (partially serves to prevent state-based statues from depriving previously enslaved Black Americans from their constitutional rights; Hoag, 2020), and 15th (right to vote; Crum, 2020) amendments have been documented and written about extensively in American history and the present day.

2.2 Black American Healthcare and Socioeconomic Disparities

Socioeconomic disparities, stemming from structural racism, have profoundly impacted the Black American demographic. Research has shown that Jim Crow had long-term effects on the economic progress of Black Americans (Althoff & Reichardt, 2024). Black American families who remained enslaved till the Civil War had substantially less social and economic resources. Black Americans make up 13.6 of the US population (US Census Bureau, n.d.); however, as evidenced by the statistics located in Table 2.1, Black Americans are disproportionately represented in a number of negative healthcare and socioeconomic outcomes. Although micro, individual-level attributions have often been made for actual or perceived Black disparities (take, for example, the 1980s cocaine epidemic; Alexander, 2010; Kim et al., 2020) in America, a more logical and plausible explanation is provided by structural or macro forces that were discussed at the outset of this chapter. The specific Black disparities are nested within various healthcare and socioeconomic categories. These categories consist of addiction, education, family, financial, housing, legal, medical, occupational, and mental health domains. These categories are also of relevance because, in each of these categories, healthcare and human service professionals (social work, psychology, psychiatry, counseling, marriage and

Table 2.1 US Black, healthcare, and socioeconomic disparities

Healthcare and socioeconomic issues	Black American disparity	Source
Addiction		
Buprenorphine for OUD	Relative to Whites, Blacks were 73% less likely to get buprenorphine	Lagisetty et al., 2019
MOUD receipt	For Blacks, receipt of MOUD[a] was lowest after high-risk index events	Barnett et al., 2023
Overdose death rates	Overdose death rates increased 44% for Black Americans	CDC, 2022a
Opioid overdose deaths	Opioid overdose deaths of Black Americans exceed those of Whites	Furr-Holden et al., 2021
Education		
Suspensions	10% of Black students were suspended, relative to 2.5% of all other races	Gage et al., 2019
Family		
Child physical abuse Rpt.	Overrepresentation of Black youth in CPA reports for 44/51 US states/terr	Luken et al., 2021
Substantiated child abuse Rpt.	Poor Black children > substantiated child abuse reports, relative to Whites	Briggs et al., 2022
Financial		
Income	Black median household income was $30,619 < their White counterparts	USCB, 2020
Poverty	Blacks Americans in poverty was 1.8 > than the general US population	USCB, 2020
Wealth	Black and White families, the median wealth was 24 k and 188 k, respectively	BGFRS, 2020
Housing		
Environmental injustice	Black Americans, ≥ 65 y/o, explained 25% of all air-pollution mortality[b]	Spiller et al., 2021
Homeownership	Black early adults have a 59% lower odds of homeownership	Modi & Sewell, 2022
Legal		
Incarceration: Jail	Of the individuals in local jails, 35% were Black[c]	BJS, 2022
Incarceration: Prison	Blacks had the highest imprisonment rate at 1186/100k[c]	BJS, 2022
Police killings: Men	Black men, 2.5 x more likely to be killed by police than White men	Edwards et al., 2019
Police killings: Women	Black women,1.4 x more likely to be killed by police than White women	Edwards et al., 2019
Medical		
COVID-19	The risk of COVID-19 death was greater among Black Americans[d]	Gross et al., 2020
Analgesic pain treatment	Blacks, relative to Whites, are less likely to receive analgesic tx for acute pain	Lee et al., 2019
Maternal mortality	Maternal mortality is highest in Blacks, 55.3 deaths/100 k live births	Hoyert, 2022

(continued)

Table 2.1 (continued)

Healthcare and socioeconomic issues	Black American disparity	Source
Infant mortality	Infant mortality is highest in Blacks, 10.6 deaths/1000 live births	CDC, 2022b
Emergency room visits	Blacks, relative to Whites, are more likely to use ED for a chronic issue	Parast et al., 2022
Breast cancer	Black women have highest breast cancer mortality, 40% > than Whites	DeSantis et al., 2019
Mental health		
Black suicide	Age-adjusted suicide rates for Blacks increased by 19.2%	Stone et al., 2023
Black youth suicide	Suicide rates for Black 10–24 y/o increased by 36.6%	Stone et al., 2023
Outpatient treatment	Blacks, relative to Whites, are less than half as likely to get outpatient MH tx	Olfson et al., 2023
Occupation		
Unemployment	Rates of unemployment for Blacks and Whites, 5.6 and 3.3, respectively	USBOLS, 2023

Abbreviations: BGFRS—Board of Governors of the Federal Reserve System, Bureau of Justice Statistics—BJS, CDC—Centers for Disease Control and Prevention, CPA—Child physical abuse, DCS—Department of Children Services, ED—Emergency department—Thousand, OUD—Opioid use disorder, MOUD—Medications for opioid use disorder (antagonist, partial, and full agonist), MH—Mental health, Rpt.—Report, Tx—Treatment, Terr—Territories, USBOLS—United States Bureau of Labor Statistics, USCB—United States Census Bureau

[a]In addition to buprenorphine, these medications included opioid antagonists

[b]Black Americans, 65 years of age or older, only accounted for 9% of the older population

[c]Black individuals represent 13.6 of the US population (US Census Bureau, n.d.)

[d]In 22 of 28 states which reported racial data in COVID-19 mortality

family therapy, nursing, public health) provide clinical services to Black Americans throughout the United States.

2.3 Black American Disparities: Structural Attributions and Ecological Systems Theory

Table 2.1 provides a non-exhaustive overview of some relevant Black disparities that exist within these domains. These Black disparities may make the utilization cognitive-behavioral therapy (CBT) with Black American clients more complex. In the United States, there is a history of making micro-level attributions for Black healthcare and socioeconomic disparities, which are structural in nature and rooted in long-standing systemic racism. The various healthcare and socioeconomic disparities, listed in Table 2.1, do not derive from characterological flaws or moral failings of Black Americans. To the contrary, the disparities are symptoms of historical anti-Black laws, policies, and institutions that sustain the disproportionate, negative outcomes in Black Americans. With the vast amount of data documenting Black American disparities, a theoretical framework is necessary to place the data and its mechanistic impact on Black Americans in context. Ecological systems theory (Bronfenbrenner, 1977) provides a suitable explanation for how Black Americans are impacted by various nested and interacting social systems that have evolved since the Transatlantic slave trade.

Bronfenbrenner's (1977) ecological systems theory has divided the social environment into several strata: microsystem, mezzosystem, exosystem, and macrosystem. The individual's relationship with a social environment or setting has been referred to as the microsystem (domestic, occupational, educational…). The relationships among social environments that interact with the individual have been called the Mezzosystem. Factors that influence the social environments that the individual interacts with are the Exosystem (community, different levels of government, the economy, and social media). Macrosystems consist of laws, policies, structures/systems, cultural norms, and politics, from which the other aforementioned systems derive. These systems (micro through macro) will be used to briefly outline how anti-Black structural racism has created and sustained Black American disparities. Across the strata in ecological systems theory, racism and discrimination occur with a compounding effect that serves to create and enhance the disparate Black American status quo that is observed in healthcare and socioeconomic indicators. The systems are mutually interacting and dependent on one another, such that a change in one system that serves to ameliorate Black disparity can be countered or thwarted by a change in another system. This exchange or ebb and flow of pro-and anti-Black initiatives at different system levels has been historically illustrated in several ways. Take, for example, the activity of the domestic terrorist Ku Klux Klan (KKK) group (exosystem) that was chronologically linked to post-Civil War Reconstruction (macrosystem) (Alexander, 2010). The increased White supremacist and nationalistic movement (macrosystem) following growing levels of racial heterogeneity (macrosystem) in predominantly White societies (Sengupta et al., 2019) provides another exemplar.

There are four additional examples provided, which illustrate the ways in which multiple systems (micro–macro) can interact to sustain Black disparities in healthcare and socioeconomic status (SES).

Example 1

There has been intimidation, violence, and death associated with Black Americans seeking to use their 15th amendment right to vote (Santoro, 2008). The 15th amendment represents a change at the macrosystem level to address a disparity in Black voting. However, after the 15th amendment was granted, at the exosystem level, fear, violence, domestic terrorism, and murder decreased the likelihood of Black Americans voting.

Example 2

A second example is provided using the enslavement of Black individuals in America. The transatlantic slave trade provided a number of financial and psychological benefits to the United States and its free citizens (Alexander, 2010; Delgado

& Stefancic, 2023). As was previously mentioned in this chapter, the enslavement of Black Americans (although slavery was not mentioned in the US Constitution) was supported with Black enslaved individuals being counted as three-fifths of a person for taxation, representation, and the psychological satisfaction of some White southerners (Hall & Feldmeier, 2017). This constitutional upholding of slavery represented a macrosystem, foundational disparity that set the groundwork for later disparities. After the Emancipation Proclamation, the 13th amendment (a macrosystem change) made slavery unconstitutional unless it was for imprisonment, another later macrosystem change. Subsequent changes at the exosystem level (police arrests), leading to mass incarceration of Black individuals have since reinstated the imprisonment of Black individuals as well as a removal of rights (Alexander, 2010). The third example incorporates micro, mezzo, and macro systems, as they pertain to disparities in education.

Example 3
The separate but equal legal doctrine from the US supreme court (Mohamed, 2022) represented macrosystem support for the legal segregation of races in America in various public settings or mezzosystems. This ruling was later overturned and found to violate the 14th amendment (another macro change). This demonstrates the ebb and flow where one macrosystem-level change trumped another to address various Black disparities in education and other mezzosystems. However, it has been argued that due to intergenerational drag (Margo, 1990), even if the segregated facilities or mezzosystem-level settings were equal, Black children would have still been at a substantial disparity between Black and White children because at the family level (microsystem), lower SES and high illiteracy would have thwarted narrowing of the educational disparities.

Example 4
A final example considers disparities in Black Americans healthcare. While the passing of the Affordable Care Act (macrosystem changes) has expanded access to healthcare providers (Buchmueller & Levy, 2020), implicit bias toward Black Americans (Kalata et al., 2022) at the mezzosystem level may ultimately discourage Black Americans from using psychotherapy or preventative medicine, which has been afforded at the macrosystem level. These implicit bias factors, associated with healthcare providers, at the mezzosystem level, may increase Black American disproportionate use of emergency departments for medical (Parast et al., 2022) and psychiatric emergencies (Peters et al., 2023). These multiple systems (micro, mezzo, exo, and macro) each provide their own contributions to and counterbalance for corrective efforts regarding Black American disparities. Due to the widespread and profound Black American disparities at each of the levels in ecological systems theory, there is a Black translatory distrust of systems/structures, that remains regardless of the potential benefit of the medical intervention/prevention (COVID-19 vaccine), civic behavior (voting, jury duty), service (healthcare), and research endeavor that is offered by the respective system (institution and policy). This Black distrust of systems can amplify the categorical disparities in Table 2.1.

2.4 The Nexus Between Structural Racism and Black American Mental Health

Black disparities are rooted in structural racism that has evolved over decades, and the individual, micro-level impacts are profound. The broader macro system and its subsidiary levels (mezzosystem and ecosystem) have fundamental impacts on individual and collective, Black mental health. This deleterious impact of anti-Black racism and discrimination can be seen in various forms of worsening Black mental health (Cavalhieri et al., 2023; Desai et al., 2023), Black trauma (Gregory Jr. & Tucker Edmonds, 2023; Spann, 2022), and internalized racism (Mouzon & McLean, 2017). As it pertains to the structural context of CBT with Black Americans, issues of racism, discrimination, Black trauma, and internalized racism are necessary considerations given their systemic catalysts. Any Black American client may come to a CBT session with none or all of these issues present. Depending on the Black client's diagnosis, unique attributes, and the clinician's skill level, all or none of these issues may be pertinent to the treatment plan. Due to the substantive historical and contemporary impact of racism and discrimination and Black trauma, meaningful discussions of CBT with Black Americans may include and address these topics.

2.4.1 Racism and Discrimination: The Impact on Black Mental Health

The effects of racism and discrimination have been studied using various methods. An earlier meta-analysis found that there was a small, positive relationship between perceived racism and its associations with Black individuals experiencing depression/anxiety, symptoms of mental illness, life satisfaction, and overall distress (Pieterse et al., 2023). This means that as perceived racism increased, each of the aforementioned four indicators of mental illness increased as well. More recent meta-analytic research has shown that there is a small, yet statistically significant, positive relationship between racial discrimination and Black mental illness (Carter & Muchow, 2017). Therefore, as racial discrimination increased, mental health distress also increased in Black individuals. Cavalhieri et al. (2023) examined the effect of online and institutional racism on symptoms of mental illness in Black individuals. The study showed significant relationships indicating that as online racism increased, symptoms of mental illness worsened, and the well-being of the participants decreased. The relationship between racism/discrimination and Black mental health has been substantively explored via qualitative studies as well. The qualitative research on the mental health impact of racism and discrimination provides granular-level details of the lived experiences of Black Americans. The study conducted by Desai and associates (2023), documented some of the emotionally painful and psychologically jarring effects of racism and discrimination stemming from police brutality, race-related occupational difficulties, and disparities in policy responses to racialized drug issues. Gregory and associates (Gregory Jr. et al., in press) structural equation model empirically showed a linear relationship between Black men's Tripartite Police Fear and increased perceived cultural barriers to obtaining mental health treatment.

2.4.2 *Black Trauma*

From the Transatlantic slave trade to the widely disseminated public murder of George Floyd, structural, institutional, and interpersonal racism includes a history of traumatic events for Black American individuals, families, and communities. These race-based traumatic events have been referred to as ethno-racial trauma (Chavez-Dueñas et al., 2019). Ethno-racial trauma consists of personal or group-based, psychological harm and apprehension, stemming from an experience with threats or danger directed to racial or ethnic minorities. Various forms of Black trauma have been identified in the behavioral and social science literature, including cultural (Alexander, 2016), historical and intergenerational trauma (Mohatt et al., 2014). Cultural trauma (Alexander, 2016) involves members of a shared group, collectively believing they experienced a dreadful or appalling event that permanently changes the group's memory and prospective identity. While the murder of George Floyd is a recent epitome of cultural trauma, other prominent examples include the killing of Emmett Till in 1955 and the infamous beating of Rodney King in 1991. Based on the definition of cultural trauma, formal state and federal criminal trials that function to provide justice for anti-Black traumatic events in America, which are collectively perceived as ultimately yielding no tangible forms of justice (by many Black Americans), could arguably also be called examples of cultural trauma (Gregory Jr. & Tucker Edmonds, 2023). Defining features of historical trauma include a group of individuals (in the context of the present book, Black Americans) experiencing some horrendous event (slavery), and the symptoms of that terrible event are continued across subsequent generations who were not present for the initial trauma. According to Mohatt and colleagues, intergenerational trauma includes the same characteristics of historical trauma; however, in intergenerational trauma, the traumatic symptoms are transmitted at the family level, rather than a group level.

2.4.3 *Internalized Anti-Black Racism*

Pyke (2010) has provided a very useful and multifaceted overall definition of internalized racism. Pyke's definition of internalized racism can be amended to more specifically define anti-Black internalized racism. Internalized anti-Black racism is the Black individual's covert or overt adoption of negative, stereotypical, Black-denigrating beliefs about themselves and/or their Black race/culture. Internalized anti-Black racism can result in emotional distress and interpersonal dysfunction.

Despite its micro-level psychosocial consequences, internalized anti-Black racism is inherently linked to and sustained by broader structural and social forces. Internalized racism has been considered as possibly the worst psychological consequence of racism (Speight, 2007). A meta-analysis consisting of predominantly Black participants showed internalized racism was positively correlated with negative mental and physical health outcomes (Gale et al., 2020). These correlations were both small and statistically significant. It is noteworthy that the correlation between internalized racism and negative mental health outcomes was significantly greater than the correlation between internalized racism and negative physical health outcomes.

2.5 Black American Strength and Resilience despite Structural Racism

To be clear, chattel slavery, Black Codes, Jim Crow, mass incarceration, socioeconomic inequity, and health disparities are in no way indicative of Black American attributes or characteristics. However, these factors are indicative of structural racism, which Black Americans have encountered in various forms since arriving in the United States. It is important that readers not conflate Black American individuals and culture with human atrocities that Black Americans have experienced in the United States. The sum of structural racism (anti-Black laws, policies, institutions, etc.) and its negative biopsychosocial sequalae are only part of the story of Black Americans; the other part of the story is the consistent psychological, social, and biological strength and resilience that's been demonstrated by Black Americans in response to these stressors (Taylor Jr et al., 2020). Black American history shows a consistent theme of effective post-US construction era responses to evolving forms of anti-Black structural racism. Historically Black Colleges and Universities have increased the educational attainment of Black Americans since slavery ended (Noonan et al., 2016). In 2005, Kaba discussed educational progress that had been obtained by Black Americans from the 1970s to the twenty-first century. In his review of educational attainment research, Kaba discussed educational advancements made by Black Americans and the impact it has on income and wealth. Kaba noted that Black men have less educational attainment than their Black female counterparts. Black progress in the United States has also been demonstrated in positive changes in federal laws and/or legislation (1954: Brown vs Board of Education; 1964–1969: Civil Rights Act, Fair Housing Act, Affirmative Action) and the election of a Black president to the highest office (Rigueur & Beshlian, 2019). The Patient Protection and Affordable Care Act was considered beneficial in expanding access to healthcare for Black Americans (Noonan et al., 2016). Yet, it should be noted that Noonan and associates and Rigueur and Beshlian constantly reiterate the tendency for Black progress to be frustrated and suffer drawbacks in the United States. In congruence with this sentiment, research has suggested that White individuals in America may assume that Black socioeconomic equality is currently achieved presently and minimize the extent of socioeconomic disparities in the past (Onyeador et al., 2021). For the purposes of this chapter and book, it is important to note that despite structural racism, the resilience and strength of Black Americans continue and progress has been achieved. Yet, as evidenced by the disparities in Table 2.1 there is still much social change that needs to occur. The historical, contemporary, idiosyncratic, and collective strengths and resilience of Black Americans can be mobilized to advance mental health outcomes.

2.6 The Structural Basis of Black American Disparities: Implications for Cognitive-Behavioral Therapy

There are a number of reasons for cognitive-behavioral clinicians to be aware of the structural roots of Black American disparities. Knowledge and comprehension of the structural basis for Black disparities will aid in:

1. Understanding the macro or upstream causes of Black trauma.
2. Developing and maintaining therapeutic rapport which could be threatened by implicit bias (Gran-Ruaz et al., 2022).
3. Creating case conceptualizations that are comprehensive and indicative of diverse Black American lived experiences.
4. Applying cognitive-behavioral interventions in precise ways to address intrapersonal, interpersonal, and environmental coping that is relevant to treatment outcomes.

A hypothetical example, using Ellis's (1994) activating event (A), beliefs about the event (B), consequences due to the belief (C), disputing the belief (D) model, is provided. A Black mother named *Serita*, came to her cognitive-behavioral therapy session with an agenda to discuss a stressful relationship with her son's teacher (A) that leaves her feeling helpless and anxious (C). The situation involves her son getting suspended (A) and *Serita* believed that the teacher was targeting her son maliciously, based on his Black race (B). First, the clinician's knowledge of structural anti-Black racism may provide some nuanced recognition of the fact that Black individuals he sees in practice live within an environment of structures and institutions which may impact his clients' diagnoses, symptoms, functioning, and goals for better or worse. Second, knowledge of anti-Black structural racism may help provide a buffer against the clinician imposing their own values of what's real or true on the Black client, thereby adding some empathy and protection for the therapeutic rapport. Third, anti-Black structural knowledge may also help the clinician to identify how his own values and experiences may contrast with those of his Black client. Fourth, in conceptualizing *Serita's* case, the clinician would include those structural, interpersonal, and intrapersonal elements which are believed to substantively impact her goals. Finally, this conceptualization, including structural and interpersonal elements, would aid in determining those aspects of *Serita's* case which are amenable to cognitive-behavioral intervention, such as cognitive restructuring and problem-solving, and those aspects which are not.

In this example, *Serita* had a fundamentally different lived experience and interpretation of those experiences than that of her clinician. The clinician first explained the cognitive model to *Serita* and she understood the cognitive model. The clinician also established a sufficient therapeutic rapport with *Serita,* which facilitates frank discussions regarding anti-Black racism. The clinician asked *Serita* questions regarding the extent to which her thought (B: "*Serita* believing that the teacher is targeting her son maliciously, based on his Black race") about the teacher was disturbing or an impediment to her (Serita) interacting with her son's teacher and ultimately addressing her son's education. *Serita* was asked if she would like to systematically consider the evidence supporting her belief about her son's teacher (D). *Serita,* having understood the cognitive model, wished to evaluate her thought using the cognitive restructuring exercise. The clinician believed that the intervention would have therapeutic benefit, whether the thought was ultimately supported by the evidence or not. After the evaluation, Serita concluded that her thoughts regarding her son's teacher were supported by the evidence. The clinician worked with Serita on problem-solving for what practical steps could be taken to address her concerns about her son's education and alleviate stress associated with the situation. Both in session and homework, Serita was also taught to use cognitive restructuring to cope with negative beliefs about herself, which undermined or discounted her ability to effectively respond to racially charged situations.

2.7 The Structural Context of Cognitive-Behavioral Therapy with Black Americans: Summary

In the US Black Americans have unique historical experiences which affect their sociology, disparities, opportunities, mental health, and the implementation of CBT. Closely related to the truth of Black American history and the CBT process, unique historical contributions from Africa are briefly discussed. Laws, policies, and other legal mechanisms that have contributed to sustained disparities in socioeconomic status, physical, and mental health were discussed. The implications of structural anti-Black racism for CBT are provided. Given its association with structural racism and potential impact on therapy, implicit bias (Galvan & Payne, 2024) and its implications for cognitive-behavioral clinicians are discussed in Chap. 3.

References

Alexander, J. C. (2016). Culture trauma, morality and solidarity. *Thesis Eleven, 132*(1), 3–16. https://doi.org/10.1177/0725513615625239

Alexander, M. (2010). *The new Jim crow: Mass incarceration in the ages of colorblindness*. The New Press.

Althoff, L., & Reichardt, H. (2024). Jim crow and black economic Progress after slavery*. *Quarterly Journal of Economics, 139*(4), 2279–2330. https://doi.org/10.1093/qje/qjae023

Barnett, M. L., Meara, E., Lewinson, T., Hardy, B., Chyn, D., Onsando, M., Huskamp, H. A., Mehrotra, A., & Morden, N. E. (2023). Racial inequality in receipt of medications for opioid use disorder. *The New England Journal of Medicine, 388*(19), 1779–1789. https://doi.org/10.1056/NEJMsa2212412

Beermann, J. M. (2020). Crisis? Whose crisis? *William & Mary Law Review, 61*(4), 931–969. https://scholarship.law.wm.edu/wmlr/vol61/iss4/2

Board of Governors of the Federal Reserve System. (2020, September 28). Disparities in wealth by race and ethnicity in the 2019 Survey of Consumer Finances. https://www.federalreserve.gov/econres/notes/feds-notes/disparities-in-wealth-by-race-and-ethnicity-in-the-2019-survey-of-consumer-finances-20200928.html

Briggs, H. E., Huggins-Hoyt, K. Y., Teasley, M. L., & Hopps, J. G. (2022). Poverty or racism?: Determinants of disproportionality and disparity for African American/black children in child welfare. *Research on Social Work Practice, 32*(5), 533–538. https://doi.org/10.1177/10497315221076830

Bronfenbrenner, U. (1977). Toward an experimental ecology of human development. *American Psychologist, 32*(7), 513–531. https://doi.org/10.1037/0003-066X.32.7.513

Buchmueller, T. C., & Levy, H. G. (2020). The ACA'S impact on racial and ethnic disparities in health insurance coverage and access to care. *Health Affairs, 39*(3), 395–402. https://doi.org/10.1377/hlthaff.2019.01394

Bureau of Justice Statistics. (2022, December 20). U.S. jail population increased while prison population decreased in 2021. https://bjs.ojp.gov/sites/g/files/xyckuh236/files/media/document/p21st_ji21st_prB.pdf

Carter, R. T., & Muchow, C. (2017). Construct validity of the race-based traumatic stress symptom scale and tests of measurement equivalence. *Psychological Trauma Theory Research Practice and Policy, 9*(6), 688–695. https://doi.org/10.1037/tra0000256

Cavalhieri, K. E., Greer, T. M., Hawkins, D., Choi, H., Hardy, C., & Heavner, E. (2023). The effects of online and institutional racism on the mental health of African Americans. *Cultural Diversity and Ethnic Minority Psychology, 30*(3), 476–486. https://doi.org/10.1037/cdp0000585

Centers for Disease Control and Prevention. (2022a, July 19). Overdose deathrates increase significantly for Black, American Indiana/Alaska native people in 2020. https://www.cdc.gov/media/releases/2022/s0719-overdose-rates-vs.html#:~:text=Opioid%20overdose%20rates%20in%202020,16)%20people%20per%20100%2C000

Centers for Disease Control and Prevention. (2022b, June 22). Infant mortality. https://www.cdc.gov/reproductivehealth/maternalinfanthealth/infantmortality.htm#print

Chavez-Dueñas, N. Y., Adames, H. Y., Perez-Chavez, J. G., & Salas, S. P. (2019). Healing ethnoracial trauma in Latinx immigrant communities: Cultivating hope, resistance, and action. *American Psychologist, 74*(1), 49–62. https://doi.org/10.1037/amp0000289

Crum, T. (2020). Reconstructing racially polarized voting. *Duke Law Journal, 70*(2), 261–331.

Delgado, R., & Stefancic, J. (2023). *Critical race theory: An introduction* (4th ed.). New York University Press.

Desai, M. U., Guy, K., Brown, M., Thompson, D., Manning, B., Johnson, S., Davidson, L., & Bellamy, C. (2023). "That was a state of depression by itself dealing with society": Atmospheric racism, mental health, and the black and African American faith community. *American Journal of Community Psychology, 73*(1–2), 104–117. https://doi.org/10.1002/ajcp.12654

DeSantis, C. E., Ma, J., Gaudet, M. M., Newman, L. A., Miller, K. D., Goding Sauer, A., Jemal, A., & Siegel, R. L. (2019). Breast cancer statistics, 2019. *CA: A Cancer Journal for Clinicians, 69*(6), 438–451. https://doi.org/10.3322/caac.21583

Edwards, F., Lee, H., & Esposito, M. (2019). Risk of being killed by police use of force in the United States by age, race-ethnicity, and sex. *Proceedings of the National Academy of Sciences of the United States of America, 116*(34), 16793–16798. https://doi.org/10.1073/pnas.1821204116

Ellis, A. (1994). *Reason and emotion in psychotherapy: A comprehensive method of treating human disturbances (revised and updated).* Carol Publishing Group.

Furr-Holden, D., Milam, A. J., Wang, L., & Sadler, R. (2021). African Americans now outpace whites in opioid-involved overdose deaths: a comparison of temporal trends from 1999 to 2018. *Abstract Addiction, 116*(3), 677–683. https://doi.org/10.1111/add.v116.3 10.1111/add.15233

Gage, N. A., Whitford, D. K., Katsiyannis, A., Adams, S., & Jasper, A. (2019). National Analysis of the disciplinary exclusion of black students with and without disabilities. *Journal of Child and Family Studies, 28*(7), 1754–1764. https://doi.org/10.1007/s10826-019-01407-7

Gale, M. M., Pieterse, A. L., Lee, D. L., Huynh, K., Powell, S., & Kirkinis, K. (2020). A meta-analysis of the relationship between internalized racial oppression and health-related outcomes. *The Counseling Psychologist, 48*(4), 498–525. https://doi.org/10.1177/0011000020904454

Galvan, M. J., & Payne, B. K. (2024). Implicit bias as a cognitive manifestation of systemic racism. *Daedalus: Journal of the American Academy of Arts & Sciences, 153*(1), 106–122. https://doi-org.proxy.ulib.uits.iu.edu/10.1162/daed_a_02051

Gibbons, A. (2017). Oldest members of our species discovered in Morocco. *Science, 356*(6342), 993–994. https://doi.org/10.1126/science.356.6342.993

Gran-Ruaz, S., Feliciano, J., Bartlett, A., & Williams, M. T. (2022). Implicit racial bias across Ethnoracial groups in Canada and the United States and black mental health. *Canadian Psychology, 63*(4), 608–622. https://doi.org/10.1037/cap0000323

Gregory, V. L., Jr., & Clary, K. L. (2022). Addressing anti-black racism: The roles of social work. *Smith College Studies In Social Work, 92*(1), 1–27. https://doi.org/10.1080/00377317.2021.2008287

Gregory, V. L., Jr., Miller, B. L., & Lipsey, A. (in press). Black men, structural racism, cultural barriers: Structural equation model with cognitive-behavioral implications. *The Counseling Psychologist.*

Gregory, V. L., Jr., & Tucker Edmonds, J. L. (2023). The racial pandemic experienced by black American men: Cognitive-behavioral and structural implications. *American Journal of Orthopsychiatry, 93*(1), 1–16. https://doi.org/10.1037/ort0000651

Gross, C. P., Essien, U. R., Pasha, S., Gross, J. R., Wang, S.-Y., & Nunez-Smith, M. (2020). Racial and ethnic disparities in population-level Covid-19 mortality. *Journal of General Internal Medicine, 35*(10), 3097–3099. https://doi.org/10.1007/s11606-020-06081-w

Hall, D. E., & Feldmeier, J. P. (2017). *Constitutional law: Governmental powers and individual freedoms* (3rd ed.). Pearson.

Hasbrouck, B. (2021). The unconstitutional police. *Harvard Civil Rights-Civil Liberties Law Review, 56*(2), 239–266.

Hoag, A. (2020). Valuing black lives: A case for ending the death penalty. *Columbia Human Rights Law Review, 51*(3), 983–1007.

Hoyert, D. L. (2022). Maternal mortality rates in the United States, 2020. *National Center for Health Statistics Health E-Stats., 71*(15), 11. https://doi.org/10.15620/cdc:113967

Jackson, J. G. (2017). *Ethiopia & the origins of civilization.* Martino Fine Books.

Kagan, M. (2018). The public defender's pin: Untangling free speech regulation in the courtroom. *Northwestern University Law Review, 112*(5), 1245–1258.

Kalata, M., Kalata, K., Yen, H., Khorshid, A., Davis, T., & Meredith, J. (2022). Community perspectives on the racial disparity in perinatal outcomes. *The Journal of Maternal-Fetal & Neonatal Medicine, 35*(13), 2512–2517. https://doi.org/10.1080/14767058.2020.1786525

Kim, J. W., Morgan, E., & Nyhan, B. (2020). Treatment versus punishment: Understanding racial inequalities in drug policy. *Journal of Health Politics, Policy and Law, 45*(2), 177–209. https://doi.org/10.1215/03616878-8004850

Koester, M. (2021). The jury is still out: How Kentucky's felon exclusion statutes violate Batson and the sixth amendment. *George Mason University Civil Rights Law Journal, 31*(3), 289–309.

Lagisetty, P. A., Ross, R., Bohnert, A., Clay, M., & Maust, D. T. (2019). Buprenorphine treatment divide by race/ethnicity and payment. *JAMA Psychiatry, 76*(9), 979–981. https://doi.org/10.1001/jamapsychiatry.2019.0876

Lee, P., Le Saux, M., Siegel, R., Goyal, M., Chen, C., Ma, Y., & Meltzer, A. C. (2019). Racial and ethnic disparities in the management of acute pain in US emergency departments: Meta-analysis and systematic review. *American Journal of Emergency Medicine, 37*(9), 1770–1777. https://doi.org/10.1016/j.ajem.2019.06.014

Luken, A., Nair, R., & Fix, R. L. (2021). On racial disparities in child abuse reports: Exploratory mapping the 2018 NCANDS. *Child Maltreatment, 26*(3), 267–281. https://doi.org/10.1177/1077559521 1001926

Margo, R. A. (1990). *Race and schooling in the south, 1880–1950: An economic history*. The University of Chicago Press.

M'baye, B. (2006). The Economic Political and Social Impact of the Atlantic Slave Trade on Africa. *The European Legacy, 11*(6), 607–622. https://doi.org/10.1080/10848770600918091

Miller, K. E. (2020). The eighth amendment power to discriminate. *Washington Law Review, 95*(2), 809–867.

Modi, R., & Sewell, A. A. (2022). Unequal early adulthoods: Racial and ethnic wealth disparities during the great recession. *Sociological Quarterly, 63*(1), 21–47. https://doi.org/10.1080/00380253.2020.1865115

Mohamed, A. N. (2022). Influence of the supreme court's Plessy v. Ferguson decision on southern editorial arguments during the "massive resistance" to integration: Perspective from Alabama. *Howard Journal of Communications, 33*(3), 281–296. https://doi.org/10.1080/10646175.2021.1985660

Mohatt, N. V., Thompson, A. B., Thai, N. D., & Tebes, J. K. (2014). Historical trauma as public narrative: A conceptual review of how history impacts present-day health. *Social Science & Medicine, 106*, 128–136. https://doi.org/10.1016/j.socscimed.2014.01.043

Mouzon, D. M., & McLean, J. S. (2017). Internalized racism and mental health among African-Americans, US-born Caribbean blacks, and foreign-born Caribbean blacks. *Ethnicity & Health, 22*(1), 36–48. https://doi.org/10.1080/13557858.2016.1196652

Noonan, A. S., Velasco-Mondragon, H. E., & Wagner, F. A. (2016). Improving the health of African Americans in the USA: An overdue opportunity for social justice. *Public Health Reviews (2107–6952), 37*(1), 1–20. https://doi.org/10.1186/s40985-016-0025-4

O'Leary, M. (2021). When bonds turn to badges. *The Georgetown Law Journal, 110*(2), 404–443.

Olfson, M., Zuvekas, S. H., McClellan, C., Wall, M. M., Hankerson, S. H., & Blanco, C. (2023). Racial-ethnic disparities in outpatient mental health Care in the United States. *Psychiatric Services (Washington, D.C.), 74*(7), 674–683. https://doi.org/10.1176/appi.ps.20220365

Onyeador, I. N., Daumeyer, N. M., Rucker, J. M., Duker, A., Kraus, M. W., & Richeson, J. A. (2021). Disrupting beliefs in racial Progress: Reminders of persistent racism Alter perceptions of past, but not current, racial economic equality. *Personality and Social Psychology Bulletin, 47*(5), 753–765. https://doi.org/10.1177/0146167220942625

Parast, L., Mathews, M., Martino, S., Lehrman, W. G., Stark, D., & Elliott, M. N. (2022). Racial/ethnic differences in emergency department utilization and experience. *JGIM: Journal of General Internal Medicine, 37*(1), 49–56. https://doi.org/10.1007/s11606-021-06738-0

Peters, Z. J., Santo, L., Davis, D., & DeFrances, C. J. (2023). Emergency department visits related to mental health disorders among adults, by race and Hispanic ethnicity: United States, 2018—2020. *National Health Statistics Reports, 181*, 1–8. https://www.cdc.gov/nchs/data/nhsr/nhsr181.pdf

Pieterse, A. L., Roberson, K. L., Garcia, R., & Carter, R. T. (2023). Racial discrimination and trauma symptoms: Further support for the race-based traumatic stress symptom scale. *Cultural Diversity and Ethnic Minority Psychology, 29*(3), 332–338. https://doi.org/10.1037/cdp0000544

Pyke, K. D. (2010). What is internalized racial oppression and why don't we study it? Acknowledging racism's hidden injuries. *Sociological Perspectives, 53*(4), 551–572. https://doi.org/10.1525/sop.2010.53.4.551

Rigueur, L. W., & Beshlian, A. (2019). The history and Progress of black citizenship. *Du Bois Review: Social Science Research on Race, 16*(1), 267–277. https://doi.org/10.1017/S1742058X19000158

Santoro, W. A. (2008). The civil rights movement and the right to vote: Black protest, segregationist violence and the audience. *Social Forces, 86*(4), 1391–1414.

Sengupta, N. K., Osborne, D., & Sibley, C. G. (2019). On the psychological function of nationalistic "Whitelash.". *Political Psychology, 40*(4), 759–775. https://doi.org/10.1111/pops.12563

Slave, V. (2021). *Trans-Atlantic slave trade – estimates*. https://www.slavevoyages.org/assessment/estimates

Spann, D. (2022). Ethical considerations for psychologists addressing racial trauma experienced by black Americans. *Ethics & Behavior, 32*(2), 99–109. https://doi.org/10.1080/10508422.2021.1964080

Speight, S. L. (2007). Internalized racism: One more piece of the puzzle. *The Counseling Psychologist, 35*(1), 126–134. https://doi.org/10.1177/0011000006295119

Spiller, E., Proville, J., Roy, A., & Muller, N. Z. (2021). Mortality risk from PM2.5: A comparison of Modeling approaches to identify disparities across racial/ethnic groups in policy outcomes. *Environmental Health Perspectives, 129*(12), 127004–127012. https://doi.org/10.1289/EHP9001

Stone, D. M., Mack, K. A., & Qualters, J. (2023). Notes from the field: Recent changes in suicide rates, by race and ethnicity and age group—United States, 2021. *Morbidity and Mortality Weekly Report, 72*, 160–162. https://doi.org/10.15585/mmwr.mm7206a4

Taylor, H. A., Jr., Washington-Plaskett, T., & Quyyumi, A. A. (2020). Black resilience–broadening the narrative and the science on cardiovascular health and disease disparities. *Ethnicity & Disease, 30*(2), 365–368. https://doi.org/10.18865/ed.30.2.365

The Ancient Kemetic Roots of Library and Information Science. (2018). *Journal of Pan African Studies, 11*(4), 16–43.

United States Bureau of Labor Statistics. (2023, June 2). Table A-2. Employment status of the civilian population by race, sex, and age. https://www.bls.gov/news.release/empsit.t02.htm

United States Census Bureau. (2020, September 15). Inequalities persist despite decline in for all major race and Hispanic origin groups. https://www.census.gov/library/stories/2020/09/poverty-rates-for-blacks-and-hispanics-reached-historic-lows-in-2019.html

United States Census Bureau. (n.d.). Quick facts United States. https://www.census.gov/quickfacts/fact/table/US/RHI225221

United States Senate. (n.d.). Constitution of the United States. https://www.senate.gov/civics/constitution_item/constitution.htm#amdt_1_(1791).

Part II
Cognitive-Behavioral Principles for and Interventions with Black Americans

Chapter 3
Cognitive-Behavioral Therapy and Implicit Racial Bias

3.1 Defining Implicit Bias

One simple definition of implicit bias is a partial behavior or preference that an individual is not aware of (Gawronski et al., 2022). Implicit bias was a term that came from psychology and was used to describe psychological associations between race and other diverse human characteristics, which may lead to different judgments or actions toward members of a diverse group (Greenwald et al., 2022). Implicit bias has been contextualized as psychological heuristics or rules of thumb that enable individuals to immediately respond to stimuli (Stamps, 2021). Kahneman (2011) wrote about System 1 and 2 thinking. System 1 is very quick and automatic, while System 2 is slower, more calculated, and considerate in decision-making and action. Kahneman discusses the benefits of System 1 and acknowledges the inherent dangers associated with System 1 as well. System 1 thinking is conceptually related to implicit bias.

Much attention has been paid to implicit bias over the recent years by psychologists (Gottfried & Mulay, 2023), social workers (Bussey et al., 2022), legal professionals (Gravett, 2017a, 2017b), medical professionals (Chadwick & Baruah, 2020; Ennis, 2022), and the lay public (Greenwald et al., 2022). With the shared interests of various professions and the general public, much substantive research has been conducted regarding implicit bias. The accumulation of implicit bias research has led to systematic reviews and meta-analytic examinations pertaining to persons with a disability (Antonopoulos et al., 2023) and Black individuals (Ahadinezhad et al., 2022). Research was also conducted that involved the development (Greenwald et al., 1998) and meta-analytic evaluations of the Implicit Association Test (IAT; Greenwald et al., 2009). The IAT has been shown to be adept at evaluating stereotypical associations and having some robustness to social desirability bias or attempts to obscure bias (Greenwald et al., 1998). The meta-analysis by Greenwald and colleagues found: the average predictive validity of the IAT was moderate and

V. L. Gregory, Jr., *Cognitive-Behavioral Therapy with Black Americans*,
https://doi.org/10.1007/978-3-032-01666-9_3

compared to self-report measures the IAT had greater predictive validity with regard to racial behavior. The IAT has been used in many studies to evaluate implicit bias.

3.2 Implicit Racial Bias as a Derivative of Structural Racism

Implicit racial bias has been viewed as individual-level perspectives (Payne & Hannay, 2021). However, research has provided some support for the notion that implicit bias is influenced by the higher-order social environment (Galvan & Payne, 2024). According to Galvan and Payne, structural racism, by virtue of its historical basis, institutions, and cultural patterns, has constructed a social environment that buttresses and sustains implicit bias. In Chap. 2, the ability of anti-Black structural racism to substantively influence various levels of society was explained using Bronfenbrenner's ecological systems theory (1977). Galvan and Payne cite many of the historical and legal features of American society that were identified in Chap. 2 (chattel slavery, Black Codes, Jim Crow, 13th Amendment, racial disparity that is common, repeated occurrences of structural inequity) as contributing to implicit bias that is present today. According to Galvan and Payne, implicit biases are cognitive structures which influence behavior. This model of viewing implicit racial bias should be familiar to cognitive-behavioral clinicians because it is essentially the cognitive model (Beck, 2021).

3.3 Implicit Bias: Black Medical and Mental Health Outcomes

A systematic review examining implicit bias and healthcare professions found that healthcare providers have implicit bias that resembles broader society, and implicit bias is inversely related to healthcare quality (FitzGerald & Hurst, 2017). More specifically, implicit bias has been associated with negative outcomes pertaining to Black maternal mortality (Montalmant & Ettinger, 2024), decreased desire to use healthcare services (Armstrong-Mensah et al., 2023), and having a potential negative influence on care among Black patients with long COVID (Bergmans et al., 2024). Similar to medicine, Black mental health has been considered to be negatively influenced by implicit racism (Gran-Ruaz et al., 2022). The Gran-Ruaz and associates study yielded very important findings regarding different issues pertaining to implicit bias and Black American and Canadian mental health. First, the Gran-Ruaz study found that both White and non-White American and Canadian racial groups had a high preference for White individuals compared to Black individuals. Second, the study found the most extreme mental health outcomes in Black Americans were seen in states that had the greater Black–White IAT (B-WIAT) bias scores. Finally, after accounting for suicide rates among Whites and explicit racism, implicit bias explained 11% of Black suicides among Black individuals in the study. As it pertains to mental health, implicit racism has been considered as a potential explanation for disparities in attention deficit hyperactivity disorder and conduct disorder diagnoses among Black youth (Shalaby et al., 2024).

3.4 Implicit Racial Bias and Cognitive-Behavioral Therapy: White Clinician, Black Client

A cognitive-behavioral clinician's implicit racial bias may influence many aspects of cognitive-behavioral therapy (CBT) with Black Americans. Components of CBT which could be negatively influenced by implicit racial bias include, but are not limited to, the cognitive-behavioral case conceptualization, communications to and about the Black client, diagnostic decisions, and treatment plan. As previously stated, implicit racial bias is a derivative of structural racism. Multilevel interventions are required to deconstruct structural racism. In the next chapter, one of the cognitive-behavioral principles for Black Americans speaks directly to higher-order macro changes that are necessary to address structural racism and the negative impact it has on Black Americans. In addition to necessary macro-level changes, micro-level methods can also be used to address symptoms and decrease the clinical impact of structural racism for Black Americans engaged in CBT. Therefore, addressing the language and communicative factors that stem from structural racism and hinder treatment for Black Americans, are also very worthwhile targets for improving provider-client relationships (Hagiwara et al., 2019) in CBT.

3.4.1 Cognitive-Behavioral Case Conceptualization

Cognitive-behavioral case conceptualization is a collaborative effort between the CBT clinician and the client that involves both parties working together to define and clarify the client's presenting issues (Kuyken et al., 2009). According to Kuyken and colleagues, the cognitive-behavioral case conceptualization is used to direct the CBT process. More information is provided on cognitive-behavioral case conceptualization in Chap. 5 (*Cognitive-Behavioral Case Conceptualization with Black Americans*). As the cognitive-behavioral clinician writes a Black client's case conceptualization, it is possible that the cognitive-behavioral clinician may impose his own values (that are not shared by the Black client) onto the Black client (Beck, 1976). The potential for cognitive-behavioral case conceptualizations to be negatively influenced by implicit racial bias may come from diverging socially constructed realities (Berger & Luckmann, 1966) stemming from different lived experiences of the cognitive-behavioral clinician and the Black client. If the cognitive-behavioral clinician is White the notion of what is true may vary substantively from what a Black client, who has a different lived experience, may believe is true. The potential differences in socially constructed realities may create differences in what is considered an adaptive or a maladaptive thought. Socially constructed reality and structurally informed cognitive-behavioral case conceptualizations are discussed in more detail in Chap. 5 of this text.

3.4.2 Communication with Black Clients

Research that uses providers from more medically oriented fields also offers models of implicit racial bias that may influence the communication patterns of cognitive-behavioral clinicians. The model provided by Hagiwara and others (2019) suggests that the provider's implicit racial bias contributes to verbal and nonverbal communication, which negatively impacts the client's satisfaction, trust, and ultimately behaviors related to health. In their model addressing communication and healthcare disparities, Hagiwara and colleagues reference the Norm of Reciprocity (Gouldner, 1960), which states that help will be returned when help is provided and when help is provided, the provider of help will not be harmed. Hagiwara and associates maintain that providers who use positive communications with their clients will receive positive communications from their clients, and providers who communicate negatively with their clients will receive negative communication from their clients. For the cognitive-behavioral clinician, positive language is language that demonstrates respect, kindness, and knowledge of the Black client's perspective and experience. To the contrary, negative communication would be language that demonstrates antipathy or rejection of the client and/or their perspective or experience. A negative reciprocal communicative pattern between the cognitive-behavioral clinician and the Black client could erode therapeutic rapport. Likewise, positive communicative exchanges between the client and clinician may enhance therapeutic rapport and client trust, resulting in positive client health behaviors.

3.4.3 Communication About Black Clients

Similar to expressed verbal communications to Black clients, written and verbal communications about Black clients can be influenced by implicit racial bias. Clinicians write substantial clinical notes regarding their clients, including but not limited to biopsychosocial assessments, case notes for clinical interventions, treatment plan updates, diagnostic updates, no-show records, and closing summaries, among other clinical notes. The importance of using affirming and culturally appropriate language regarding clinical notes for Black Americans demonstrates the cognitive-behavioral clinician's respect for the client. Respectful and culturally appropriate language also contributes to the likelihood that other clinicians viewing the clinical notes may have a dignified and respectful view of the Black client. A cognitive-behavioral clinician's clinical notes may influence how other clinicians perceive and treat the Black client. Black clients who are treated harshly or disrespectfully by multiple clinicians may contribute to distrust of the mental healthcare system by Black clients and discourage engagement and retention of Black clients in mental health treatment. Another reason for preventing implicit racial bias is that the Black clients may see it themselves. The Health Insurance Portability and Accountability Act (HIPAA) allows clients substantive access to their own mental health records (Brendel et al., 2004). This means that the cognitive-behavioral clinician's writings about the patient could be a source of controversy and disrupt the therapeutic alliance.

3.4.4 Diagnostic Decisions

Meta-analytic research has found Black Americans to have the highest rate of psychotic experiences among racial/ethnic groups, and Black Americans had an increased odds of a schizophrenia diagnosis relative to their White counterparts (van der Ven et al., 2024; Schwartz et al., 2019). Implicit racial bias can contribute to diagnostic errors among Black Americans, as a diagnosing clinician's stereotypical perceptions of a Black client or their culture may lead to a psychiatric misdiagnosis (Schwartz & Blankenship, 2014). The misdiagnosis of Black Americans, stemming from implicit racial bias, is important for several reasons. There is stigma attached to mental illness and a diagnosis of a psychotic disorder can lead to the stigmatization of the Black client. Diagnoses have the function of providing a specific cause, course, and treatment for a disorder (Horwitz, 2002). Improper diagnosis of Black Americans can lead to inappropriate treatments. If the Black client is not receiving appropriate treatment for their disorder, distrust for the cognitive-behavioral clinician may increase and engagement and retention may decrease.

3.4.5 Treatment Plan

Implicit racial bias can also skew the selection of cognitive-behavioral interventions for Black Americans. Similar to the way in which Black stereotypes may play a role in the diagnostic decisions (Schwartz & Blankenship, 2014), Black stereotypes stemming from implicit racial bias can also negatively bias the selection of cognitive-behavioral interventions for a Black American client. For example, if a clinician has implicit bias that Black individuals lack the cognitive capacity to think critically and self-reflect, it's plausible that the clinician may not choose to educate the Black client on the cognitive model and may not use a cognitive restructuring intervention.

3.5 Methods to Reduce Manifest Implicit Racial Bias in Cognitive-Behavioral Therapy

In discussing ways to reduce racial bias in CBT. A distinction must be made between manifest and latent racial bias. Manifest racial bias are those behaviors, statements, writings, nonverbal communications that are directly observable. Latent racial bias includes factors that are not directly observable such as attitudes, beliefs, and thoughts that are indicative of racial bias. Implicit racial bias can be manifest, where the implicit racial bias is demonstrated and observable in writings about Black Americans or microaggressive interactions with Black American clients. Implicit racism can also be latent and not directly observable, for example, long-standing stereotypical beliefs about Black Americans and/or Black American culture. The distinction between manifest and latent implicit racial bias is consistent with the stance of Galvan and Payne (2024), which states that implicit cognitive biases (latent) influence behavior (manifest).

3.5.1 Cognitive-Behavioral Case Conceptualization

There are specific ways to address the observable manifestations of implicit racial bias. For the cognitive-behavioral case conceptualization, asking the client for feedback on the case conceptualization is one way to help increase the likelihood that the theory proposed in the case conceptualization is indicative of the Black American client's thoughts, beliefs, and current circumstances. Eliciting client feedback in CBT helps build the therapeutic alliance and provides the client with the opportunity to address any issues that may be unresolved (Beck, 2021). Beyond asking the Black client for feedback on the case conceptualization, listening intently to the feedback the Black client provides, reflecting the feedback, and coming to a consensus about the incorporation of the feedback is equally important. If the Black client has questions regarding the case conceptualization, answering the questions could be an opportunity to further elaborate on the cognitive model and its implications for treatment. It should be noted that effectively engaging the Black client and being intentional about building and sustaining a strong therapeutic rapport will help with eliciting and receiving transparent feedback from the client. As it pertains to the cognitive-behavioral case conceptualization, Black American clients should also be informed that assessment is an ongoing process rather than a one-time event. Due to assessment being a process that occurs throughout the cognitive-behavioral sessions, the case formulation may also change. The case formulation, being a living document rather than a stagnant document, should be clearly discussed with Black American clients, as it may potentially mitigate concerns the Black client may have about the initial cognitive-behavioral case formulation. Clinical case staffing opportunities and clinical supervision with cognitive-behavioral clinicians who have training and clinical experience in working with Black Americans using CBT can also help with developing a cognitive-behavioral case formulation with a Black American client. The potential benefit of using the clinical wisdom available in staffing opportunities and clinical supervision is that the cognitive-behavioral clinician has access to the experience and perspectives of others who may provide clinical insight that was not initially seen by the cognitive-behavioral clinician.

3.5.2 Communication with Black Clients

Research regarding communication methods that improve the engagement or retention of racial/ethnic minorities has been conducted and holds varying degrees of relevance for CBT with Black Americans. A systematic review examined clinician communication and engagement of racial/ethnic minorities in mental health treatment (Aggarwal et al., 2016). The authors drew the following conclusions regarding improving client engagement:

- Clients' relevant perceptions of mental illness should be integrated into their treatment plan.
- Interpersonal skills should be used to improve client satisfaction.
- Available mental health services should be discussed with the clients.
- Somatic symptoms and their relation to the mental health problem should be discussed.
- Stigma should be discussed.
- Client concerns about confidentiality should be addressed.

The recommendations of the systematic review are theoretically contrary to implicit racial bias. Focusing the client's perception of mental illness centers the client's perspective rather than the clinician's or at least demonstrates some collaborative spirit. Substantive use of interpersonal skills to increase satisfaction may capitalize on Hagiwara et al.'s (2019) model, which places importance on the negative or positive reciprocal nature of provider and patient communication (Gouldner, 1960). If Black American clients are treated with respect then a respectful communicative pattern is more likely to be reciprocated. Discussing the available services may provide some degree of empowerment by presenting possible options for treatment. There has been a long-held belief that racial/ethnic minority clients report more somatic symptoms for psychological distress. However, more recent research has called this notion into question (Sauceda et al., 2021). The discussion of stigma in mental illness pertaining to Black Americans is logical given that the same structural sources that catalyzes implicit racial bias among clinicians may also sustain stigma regarding treatment for mental illness in Black communities. Discussing confidentiality may address some underlying medical or structural distrust that Black Americans may already have based on historical structural racism. This systematic review offers logical and broadly relevant information; however, the systematic review was not limited to Black Americans or CBT. Despite this, the recommendations align with some extant research. A key component in working with Black Americans using CBT would be to buttress the therapeutic alliance by demonstrating respect in verbal and nonverbal communication. Chapter 8 elucidates this topic more as CBT with Black American men and women is discussed.

3.5.3 *Communication About Black Clients*

A narrative review conducted in the field of medicine examined biased and stigmatizing language and provided recommendations for supporting health equity (Healy et al., 2022). The recommendations by Healy and associates were relevant for communications regarding Black Americans receiving cognitive-behavioral therapy for mental health treatment. The authors recommend: (1) Not conflating a client's condition with their identity by using phrases such as an individual with… rather than referring to client as the name of their disorder, for example, "a person with an alcohol use disorder," rather than an "alcoholic," (2) Referring to a client's behavior, rather than using a behavior do broadly identify the client. For example, instead of stating, "the client is aggressive," the cognitive-behavioral clinician may state, "the client raised his voice when asked what his thoughts were about the situation?" (3) Avoid discrediting clients by selectively, sarcastically, or humorously using the client's quotes. (4) Avoid placing emphasis on race that underscores the notion of biological, rather than socially constructed race. For example, leading with, "Black women with psychotic symptoms," may also place emphasis on the overdiagnosis of and stereotype of Black individuals with psychotic disorders and may undermine the fact that the psychotic symptoms may be part of a sever depressive episode. (5) Avoiding language that blames clients for their disorder or lack of recovery. (6) Avoid language that diminishes the client's reported experience.

Communications about Black American clients provides ample opportunity for the manifest expression of a clinician's implicit racial bias because the client is typically unaware of what I being written about him unless he requests to see his record. Managers and directors may have policy regarding language use regarding clients and this is also an issue that could be addressed in case staffing as well as individual or group clinical supervision. The recommendations by Healy and associates do not deal exclusively with Black Americans but instead address factors that could be written about many clients. When considered in the context of Black Americans receiving CBT for mental illness, the recommendations underscore the compounding or dual burden (Joseph et al., 2021) experienced by Black Americans when clinicians write in a biased or stigmatizing fashion about them.

3.5.4 Diagnostic Decisions

Diagnostic decisions stemming from implicit racial bias may be addressed in various ways across various levels depending on the context in which diagnostic decisions are made. For community mental health centers, that have master's level cognitive-behavioral clinicians that require a physician's signature on the diagnosis, the signing physician may play a central role in asking clinical questions that may prevent implicit racial bias from influencing the Black client's diagnosis and subsequent treatment. Questions asked by a signing physician would in essence be questions that determine if an alternative diagnosis may better explain the symptoms which are reported by the client. Schwartz et al. (2019) have discussed the possibility that diagnosing clinicians may confuse a client's speech with diagnostic symptoms. Peer consultation and clinical supervision from clinician that have diagnostic experience with Black Americans may also be good supports. Reviewing clinical research on diagnostic issues pertinent to Black Americans is also a good resource for decreasing implicit racial bias from negatively influencing the diagnostic process.

3.5.5 Treatment Plan

The choice of treatment plan interventions can be influenced by implicit racial bias. Implicit racial bias may influence a Black American client's cognitive-behavioral treatment plan in several ways. First, interventions that align with the clinician's stereotypical perceptions of the Black American client may be included. Second, interventions that are contrary to the clinician's stereotypical perception of the client may not be used. Both instances are indicative of implicit racial bias negatively influencing the Black American client's cognitive-behavioral treatment plan. Similar to the cognitive-behavioral case conceptualization, the treatment interventions should be discussed with the Black American client to determine the client's input on what interventions he thinks would be most appropriate. Questions for the Black American client regarding what interventions may have been effective in the past could be useful. The Black American client could also be given the Cognitive-Behavioral Coping Skills subscale of the CuTS (Gregory Jr. & Tucker Edmonds, 2024a, 2024b). Once he completes this subscale, the cognitive-behavioral clinician could use the client's responses to further discuss cognitive-behavioral interventions which may be useful in treatment. The 27 item and 22 item versions of the CuTS are available in Appendices C and D of this text.

3.5.6 Methods to Reduce Latent Implicit Racial Bias in Cognitive-Behavioral Therapy

In accordance with the belief that implicit racial bias is closely related to structural racism, methods for decreasing structural racism include changing the organizational norms of an agency, large policy changes, and having more racial minorities employed at high level positions (Payne & Hannay, 2021). These are changes that may occur in mental health agencies to decrease implicit racial bias among cognitive-behavioral clinicians. Micro oriented approaches with some promise were identified in a systematic review (FitzGerald et al., 2019). Studies meeting inclusion criteria for the systematic review primarily consisted of Black and White implicit racial bias. The following implicit racial bias interventions were found to be the most promising: intentional methods to overcome biases, exposure to disconfirming experiences, self-identification with the other group, and emotion induction. This systematic review included pre-experimental studies and used vote-counting, therefore it did not have the statistical precision of a meta-analysis.

3.5.7 Project Implicit: Implicit Association Test

The outcomes of the implicit bias interventions in the systematic review (FitzGerald et al., 2019) used the IAT or similar measures. For cognitive-behavioral clinicians wishing to evaluate the extent of Black implicit racial bias they may hold, as of the writing of this text, Project Implicit (2011) had a website that allowed individuals 18 years and older to complete different versions of the IAT including but not limited to race, ethnicity, gender, age, and many other demographic categories which implicit bias may exist. As it pertains to Black Americans IATs regarding race (Black–White), skin tone (Light Skin–Dark Skin), and weapons (Black and White faces regarding weapons and harmless objects) are available. The project implicit website has an Institutional Review Board contact and a caveat regarding the interpreted test results. Mental health agency managers, directors, consultants, or other appropriately trained personnel may potentially use the Project Implicit IAT to create self-awareness or insight regarding implicit anti-Black racial bias.

3.6 Implicit Racial Bias and Cognitive-Behavioral Therapy: Black Clinician, Black Client

As seen in the narrative review conducted by FitzGerald and associates (2019), considerably more research has looked at implicit racism in the context of the Black–White dynamic. Considerably less research has been conducted regarding internalized or other anti-Black racism among non-White individuals who work with Black Americans. Within the context of structural racism, it is important to consider the extent to which Black therapists may internalize negative beliefs about Black clients, culture, and themselves as Black individuals, given the potential for these internalizations to negatively impact CBT with Black American clients. Internalized anti-Black racism among Black clinicians may be especially detrimental for a number of reasons. First, given the often implicit nature of internalized anti-Black racism, the cognitive-behavioral clinician may have no or varying degrees of insight into their own anti-Black internalized racism. A Black clinician who holds anti-Black beliefs regarding the clients they serve may not be able to effectively engage, diagnose, conceptualize, treat, and/or advocate for Black American clients. The lack of insight pertaining to internalized anti-Black racism may also negatively influence family members of Black American clients who are stakeholders in the therapeutic outcomes. A Black cognitive-behavioral clinician's own implicit racial bias may negatively impact other clinicians as well as the collective work environment. While, at least in theory, supervision and various forms of intervention may potentially improve a Black clinician's internalized racism and its impact on clients, considerably more research is needed to address this often overlooked yet important topic.

3.7 Cognitive-Behavioral Therapy and Implicit Racial Bias: Summary

The present chapter examined various aspects of implicit racial bias as it pertained to cognitive-behavioral clinicians and their work with Black American clients. Clinical issues in CBT, including case conceptualizations, communications with and about Black American clients, diagnostic decisions, and treatment plans were discussed in their relationship to implicit racial bias and the cognitive-behavioral clinician. The impact of implicit racial bias was necessary to discuss before the use of cognitive-behavioral principles for Black Americans is presented. It is conceivable that a cognitive-behavioral clinician with implicit racial bias may not fully embrace the cognitive-behavioral principles for Black Americans. In the next chapter, cognitive-behavioral principles for Black Americans, denoted with the RESPPECTUS acronym, are identified and described.

References

Aggarwal, N. K., Pieh, M. C., Dixon, L., Guarnaccia, P., Alegría, M., & Lewis-Fernández, R. (2016). Clinician descriptions of communication strategies to improve treatment engagement by racial/ethnic minorities in mental health services: A systematic review. *Patient Education and Counseling, 99*(2), 198–209. https://doi.org/10.1016/j.pec.2015.09.002

Ahadinezhad, B., Khosravizadeh, O., Maleki, A., & Hashtroodi, A. (2022). Implicit racial bias among medical graduates and students by an IAT measure: A systematic review and meta-analysis. *Irish Journal of Medical Science, 191*(4), 1941–1949. https://doi.org/10.1007/s11845-021-02756-3

Antonopoulos, C. R., Sugden, N., & Saliba, A. (2023). Implicit bias toward people with disability: A systematic review and meta-analysis. *Rehabilitation Psychology, 68*(2), 121–134. https://doi.org/10.1037/rep0000493

Armstrong-Mensah, E., Rasheed, N., Williams, D., Moyer, K., Alema-Mensah, E., & Tetteh, A. K. (2023). Implicit racial bias, health care provider attitudes, and perceptions of health care quality among African American college students in Georgia, USA. *Journal of Racial and Ethnic Health Disparities, 10*(5), 2600–2612. https://doi.org/10.1007/s40615-022-01439-8

Beck, A. T. (1976). *Cognitive therapy and the emotional disorders*. Meridian.

Beck, J. S. (2021). *Cognitive behavior therapy: Basics and beyond* (3rd ed.). Guilford Press.

Berger, P. L., & Luckmann, T. (1966). *The social construction of reality: A treatise in the sociology of knowledge*. Anchor Books.

Bergmans, R. S., Chambers-Peeple, K., Yu, C., Xiao, L. Z., Wegryn-Jones, R., Martin, A., Dell'Imperio, S., Aboul-Hassan, D., Williams, D. A., Clauw, D. J., & DeJonckheere, M. (2024). "I'm still here, I'm alive and breathing": The experience of Black Americans with long COVID. *Journal of Clinical Nursing, 33*(1), 162–177. https://doi.org/10.1111/jocn.16733

Brendel, R. W., Bryan, E., & Schouten, R. (2004). HIPAA for psychiatrists. *Harvard Review of Psychiatry, 12*(3), 177–183. https://doi.org/10.1080/10673220490472436

Bronfenbrenner, U. (1977). Toward an experimental ecology of human development. *American Psychologist, 32*(7), 513–531. https://doi.org/10.1037/0003-066X.32.7.513

Bussey, S. R., Thompson, M. X., & Poliandro, E. (2022). Leading the charge in addressing racism and bias: Implications for social work training and practice. *Social Work Education, 41*(5), 907–925. https://doi.org/10.1080/02615479.2021.1903414

Chadwick, A. J., & Baruah, R. (2020). Gender disparity and implicit gender bias amongst doctors in intensive care medicine: A "disease" we need to recognise and treat. *Journal of the Intensive Care Society, 21*(1), 12–17. https://doi.org/10.1177/1751143719870469

Ennis, K. (2022). Addressing implicit bias to acknowledge the experience of under-represented in medicine colleagues and improve patient care. *International Journal of Psychiatry in Medicine, 57*(6), 541–546. https://doi.org/10.1177/00912174221125026

FitzGerald, C., & Hurst, S. (2017). Implicit bias in healthcare professionals: A systematic review. *BMC Medical Ethics, 18*. https://doi.org/10.1186/s12910-017-0179-8

FitzGerald, C., Martin, A., Berner, D., & Hurst, S. (2019). Interventions designed to reduce implicit prejudices and implicit stereotypes in real world contexts: A systematic review. *BMC Psychology, 7*, 29. https://doi.org/10.1186/s40359-019-0299-7

Galvan, M. J., & Payne, B. K. (2024). Implicit bias as a cognitive manifestation of systemic racism. *Daedalus: Journal of the American Academy of Arts & Sciences, 153*(1), 106–122. https://doi.org/10.1162/daed_a_02051

Gawronski, B., Ledgerwood, A., & Eastwick, P. W. (2022). Implicit bias ≠ bias on implicit measures. *Psychological Inquiry, 33*(3), 139–155. https://doi.org/10.1080/1047840X.2022.2106750

Gottfried, E. D., & Mulay, A. L. (2023). Comment on implicit gender bias in the clinical judgement of psychopathy and personality disorders among licensed psychologists in the USA. *Journal of Personality Assessment, 105*(6), 838–839. https://doi.org/10.1080/00223891.2023.2257310

Gouldner, A. W. (1960). The norm of reciprocity: A preliminary statement. *American Sociological Review, 25*(2), 161–178. https://doi.org/10.2307/2092623

Gran-Ruaz, S., Feliciano, J., Bartlett, A., & Williams, M. T. (2022). Implicit racial bias across ethnoracial groups in Canada and the United States and Black mental health. *Canadian Psychology/Psychologie Canadienne, 63*(4), 608–622. https://doi.org/10.1037/cap0000323

Gravett, W. H. (2017a). The myth of objectivity: Implicit racial bias and the law (part 1). *Potchefstroom Electronic Law Journal, 20*, 1–25. https://doi.org/10.17159/1727-3781/2017/v20i0a1312

Gravett, W. H. (2017b). The myth of objectivity: Implicit racial bias and the law (part 2). *Potchefstroom Electronic Law Journal, 20*, 1–25. https://doi.org/10.17159/1727-3781/2017/v20i0a1313

Greenwald, A. G., Dasgupta, N., Dovidio, J. F., Kang, J., Moss-Racusin, C. A., & Teachman, B. A. (2022). Implicit-bias remedies: Treating discriminatory bias as a public-health problem. *Psychological Science in the Public Interest, 23*(1), 7–40. https://doi.org/10.1177/15291006211070781

Greenwald, A. G., McGhee, D. E., & Schwartz, J. L. K. (1998). Measuring individual differences in implicit cognition: The implicit association test. *Journal of Personality and Social Psychology, 74*(6), 1464–1480. https://doi.org/10.1037/0022-3514.74.6.1464

Greenwald, A. G., Poehiman, T. A., Uhlrnann, E. L., & Banaji, M. R. (2009). Understanding and using the implicit association test: III. Meta-analysis of predictive validity. *Journal of Personality and Social Psychology, 97*(1), 17–41. https://doi.org/10.1037/a0015575

Gregory, V. L., Jr., & Tucker Edmonds, J. L. (2024a). Cultural trauma scale: Psychometric evaluation of Black men's beliefs, emotions, and coping. *Psychological Trauma Theory Research Practice and Policy, 16*(8), 1329–1337. https://doi.org/10.1037/tra0001607

Gregory, V. L., Jr., & Tucker Edmonds, J. L. (2024b). Cultural trauma scale (CuTS): Parsimonious principal component analysis, independent Black American male sample. *Journal of Aggression, Maltreatment & Trauma, 33*(3), 369–386. https://doi.org/10.1080/10926771.2023.2256741

Hagiwara, N., Elston Lafata, J., Mezuk, B., Vrana, S. R., & Fetters, M. D. (2019). Detecting implicit racial bias in provider communication behaviors to reduce disparities in healthcare: Challenges, solutions, and future directions for provider communication training. *Patient Education and Counseling, 102*(9), 1738–1743. https://doi.org/10.1016/j.pec.2019.04.023

Healy, M., Richard, A., & Kidia, K. (2022). How to reduce stigma and bias in clinical communication: A narrative review. *Journal of General Internal Medicine, 37*(10), 2533–2540. https://doi.org/10.1007/s11606-022-07609-y

Horwitz, A. V. (2002). *Creating mental illness*. The University of Chicago Press.

Joseph, N. T., Peterson, L. M., Gordon, H., & Kamarck, T. W. (2021). The double burden of racial discrimination in daily-life moments: Increases in negative emotions and depletion of psychosocial resources among emerging adult African Americans. *Cultural Diversity & Ethnic Minority Psychology, 27*(2), 234–244. https://doi.org/10.1037/cdp0000337

Kahneman, D. (2011). *Thinking, fast and slow*. Farrar, Straus, and Giroux.

Kuyken, W., Padesky, C. A., & Dudley, R. (2009). *Collaborative case conceptualization: Working effectively with clients in cognitive-behavioral therapy*. Guilford Press.

Montalmant, K. E., & Ettinger, A. K. (2024). The racial disparities in maternal mortality and impact of structural racism and implicit racial bias on pregnant Black women: A review of the literature. *Journal of Racial and Ethnic Health Disparities, 11*(6), 3658–3677. https://doi.org/10.1007/s40615-023-01816-x

Payne, B. K., & Hannay, J. W. (2021). Implicit bias reflects systemic racism. *Trends in Cognitive Sciences, 25*(11), 927–936. https://doi.org/10.1016/j.tics.2021.08.001

Project Implicit. (2011). *Project implicit*. https://implicit.harvard.edu/implicit/takeatest.html

Sauceda, J. A., Patel, A. R., Santiago-Rodriguez, E. I., Garcia, D., & Lechuga, J. (2021). Testing for differences in the reporting of somatic symptoms of depression in racial/ethnic minorities. *Health Education & Behavior, 48*(3), 260–264. https://doi.org/10.1177/10901981211011925

Schwartz, R. C., & Blankenship, D. M. (2014). Racial disparities in psychotic disorder diagnosis: A review of empirical literature. *World Journal of Psychiatry, 4*(4), 133–140. https://doi.org/10.5498/wjp.v4.i4.133

Schwartz, E. K., Docherty, N. M., Najolia, G. M., & Cohen, A. S. (2019). Exploring the racial diagnostic bias of schizophrenia using behavioral and clinical-based measures. *Journal of Abnormal Psychology, 128*(3), 263–271. https://doi.org/10.1037/abn0000409

Shalaby, N., Sengupta, S., & Williams, J. B. (2024). Large-scale analysis reveals racial disparities in the prevalence of ADHD and conduct disorders. *Scientific Reports, 14*(1), 1–9. https://doi.org/10.1038/s41598-024-75954-5

Stamps, D. C. (2021). Nursing leadership must confront implicit bias as a barrier to diversity in health care today. *Nurse Leader, 19*(6), 630–638. https://doi.org/10.1016/j.mnl.2021.02.004

van der Ven, E., Olino, T. M., Diehl, K., Nuñez, S. M., Thayer, G., Bridgwater, M. A., Ereshefsky, S., Musket, C., Lincoln, S. H., Rogers, R. T., Klaunig, M. J., Soohoo, E., DeVylder, J. E., Grattan, R. E., Schiffman, J., Ellman, L. M., Niendam, T. A., & Anglin, D. M. (2024). Ethnoracial risk variation across the psychosis continuum in the US: A systematic review and meta-analysis. *JAMA Psychiatry, 81*(5), 447–455. https://doi.org/10.1001/jamapsychiatry.2023.5497

Chapter 4
Cognitive-Behavioral RESPPECTUS Principles for Black Americans

4.1 Traditional Cognitive-Behavioral Principles: Congruence with Black Americans

The traditional principles of cognitive-behavioral therapy (CBT) are logical and well-delineated in a number of CBT texts (Beck, 1976, 2021; Leahy, 1996). The omnibus principles of CBT collectively speak to the intervention's structure, rapport, collaborative nature, temporal focus, and the use of psychotherapeutic techniques. One of the principles of CBT addresses its cultural adaptability (Beck, 2021). Judith Beck has stated that CBT has values that are inherently consistent with the majority culture, and CBT can be tailored to address cultural needs. Judith Beck also overtly discussed the role of cultural bias and it being a concern that cultural minority clients may bring to therapy. This principle of cultural adaptability is absolutely necessary and provides a general foundation for the need to implement CBT in culturally specific ways. However, the principle lacks guidance regarding specific things that can be done for Black Americans when using CBT. The question of "How do these traditional CBT principles relate to Black Americans?" remains unanswered.

Although not identified as a principle, in discussing the techniques of cognitive therapy, Aaron Beck (1976) explained the importance of client self-direction and warned against the imposition of the clinician's values on the client. Beck's (1976) discussion occurred in the context of what a maladaptive thought is and who defines it. Aaron Beck went on to state that a thought can typically be considered maladaptive if there is a consensus between the clinician and the client that a particular thought is harmful or impeding functioning. Although in 1976, Aaron Beck discussed this collaborative relationship independent of race and culture, his discussion is especially pertinent in the use of CBT with Black American clients today. Given the broad array of structural (Alexander, 2010), law enforcement (Carson, 2020), economic (Judge et al., 2023), and health related (Rogers et al., 2020) disparities that are prevalent in contemporary Black America (see Chap. 2), many Black

V. L. Gregory, Jr., *Cognitive-Behavioral Therapy with Black Americans*, https://doi.org/10.1007/978-3-032-01666-9_4

clients could have vastly different experiences and realities than their non-Black therapists. The potential for these cultural and ontological differences to undermine the establishment and maintenance of a sound therapeutic rapport, underscores the importance of Collaborative Empiricism (Beck, 2021) regarding what thoughts are maladaptive. Along the same lines, collaboration with and meaningful participation from clients is another principle of CBT (Beck, 2021). Cognitive-behavioral therapy's collaborative nature is of particular therapeutic value when working with Black American clients who may be struggling with various forms of social injustice and inequity. Adopting a collaborative relationship in the cognitive-behavioral therapeutic process helps to thwart the microcosmic reoccurrence of inequities that Black clients have had or may currently be experiencing. Race-based psychotherapeutic complexities potentially abound (Knight, 2013) when non-Black and Black clinicians engage with Black clients in the therapeutic process (Gurpinar-Morgan et al., 2014). Therefore, traditional CBT principles should be buttressed by additional specifications that are responsive to: historical and contemporary Black lived experiences, Black ontology, and Black within-group heterogeneity. In summary, the traditional CBT principles remain relevant for Black Americans. However, there are still aspects of the broader social environment (micro, mezzo, exo, and macro system factors [Bronfenbrenner, 1977], discussed in Chap. 2) and lived experiences that require additional principles to optimize CBT with Black Americans.

4.2 Cognitive-Behavioral Principles for Black Americans

Based on clinical research, theory, and clinical experiences gained from working with Black Americans using CBT, ten cognitive-behavioral principles have been developed. The systematic review conducted by Jacob and associates (2023) identified some of the common coping skills that Black Americans use to cope with racism. These themes included cognitive interventions, social support, problem-solving, and other strategies that are represented in the RESPPECTUS principles. These cognitive-behavioral principles were developed to make CBT more responsive to the diverse needs of Black Americans engaged in CBT. The cognitive-behavioral RESPPECTUS principles were also developed to aid cognitive-behavioral clinicians in using system 2 thinking (Kahneman, 2011; system 2 thinking was previously described in Chap. 3), regarding their clinical work with Black Americans. The ten CBT principles for Black Americans were intended to be used in harmony with one another. The principles provide substantive information regarding their potential use; however, they are still broad enough to complement manualized interventions. Given the purpose of the cognitive-behavioral principles for Black Americans, issues of anti-Black racism/discrimination and Black trauma are alluded to. These ten cognitive-behavioral principles for Black Americans are represented by the mnemonic acronym, RESPPECTUS. Table 4.1 and Appendix B provide the titles and a summary for each of the ten cognitive-behavioral principles. Each one of the cognitive-behavioral principles and their respective function(s), for cognitive-behavioral clinicians and Black American clients, is also narratively described below.

Table 4.1 Cognitive-behavioral principles for Black Americans: RESPPECTUS

Principle 1	Resilience and strength of Black Americans	
	Function:	Resilience and strengths of Black Americans principle calls for cognitive-behavioral clinicians to collaboratively and systematically identify and use the resilience and strengths of Black American clients to accomplish their treatment goals and personal aspirations
Principle 2	Empathy for Black traumatic events and stressors	
	Function:	This principle is manifested in verbal and non-erbal communicative behaviors that convey accurate and authentic understanding of Black American clients' perceptions and impacts of Black traumatic events and the structural forces which perpetuate them
Principle 3	Structural racism—Influences on presenting problems, rapport, and therapy	
	Function:	If structural factors are identified as being meaningful contributors to the presenting problem and/or the development of beliefs, these issues should be specified in the cognitive-behavioral case formulation
Principle 4	Problem-solving	
	Function:	Problem-solving is a fundamental intervention that is used to address those situations that are rooted in structural and interpersonal racism and not solely explained by errors in appraisal
Principle 5	Policy change	
	Function:	The primary function of the policy change principle, is the cognitive-behavioral clinician's understanding of and engagement in upstream-oriented activities to improve micro-level functioning for Black American clients with mental illness and addiction
Principle 6	Evaluating thoughts and beliefs	
	Function:	The primary functions of the evaluating thoughts and beliefs principle, involves cognitive restructuring in a collaborative, empathetic, and structurally informed manner, which makes constructive use of each Black client's individual and collective resilience and strength
Principle 7	Critical evaluation of clinical and other relevant research	
	Function:	Cognitive-behavioral clinicians must identify and critically evaluate the external validity, intersectionality, and overall utility of extant research literature for the Black American client(s) they are working with
Principle 8	Truth and transparency	
	Function:	The principle of truth and transparency, calls for the cognitive-behavioral clinician to proactively create a therapeutic culture of truth and transparency. This culture of truth and transparency includes not only the clinician and their interactions with clients, but also clinical supervisors and agency policy
Principle 9	Uniqueness of each black individual	
	Function:	The uniqueness of each Black individual principle, recognizes the within group diversity among Black American clients and uses Black heterogeneity to inform their work with Black clients
Principle 10	Social support's import	
	Function:	The primary function of the social support's import principle, is to promote cognitive-behavioral therapists in aiding Black American clients in engaging and sustaining social support networks that may be beneficial for addressing racial discrimination, various forms of psychological distress, and other stressors

4.2.1 *Principle 1: Resilience and Strength of Black Americans*

Resilience is a term used to exemplify an individual or group's robustness to psychological stressors (Kiesewetter & Huber, 2021). Structural racism provides a means for the resilience of Black Americans to be demonstrated (Turner et al., 2022). Theory and research regarding resilience and strengths within Black America, underscores the importance of the first cognitive-behavioral principle for Black Americans. The Black love, activism, and community (BLAC) model (Turner et al., 2022) is derived from research and theory regarding resiliency factors. The BLAC model emphasizes Black resilience that converges around four components: relationships, spirituality, identity, and active expression (Turner et al., 2022). According to Turner and associates, these four components of the BLAC model are used to explain the resilience of Black individuals who engage in activities to promote social justice. Relationships represent social connections with psychosocial benefits for Black Americans. Although briefly mentioned here, the importance and utility of relationships in CBT with Black Americans are further described in principle 10, *Social Support's Import*. Spirituality is inclusive of concepts pertaining to coping and trust in a God. Identity includes the sharing of coping skills for racial stressors as well as pride in the Black culture. Active Expression consists of participation in various forms of Black relevant art as well as civic-minded activities. As seen in studies cited throughout the description of principle 1, the BLAC model is congruent with extant, peer-reviewed literature citing many of the same concepts as resilience and strength-based factors for Black individuals who are not necessarily engaged in efforts to create Black social justice. Qualitative research conducted by Bauer et al. (2020) has shown evidence of resilience stemming from young Black men's willingness and success in handling issues on their own, yet still having an openness to consider formal mental health services. The same study also saw resilience demonstrated in various culturally oriented coping methods (enjoyable activities and prayer) and an ability to endure despite various traumas that were experienced. Similarly, Gregory Jr. and Tucker Edmonds (2023) examined Black male experiences with cultural trauma stemming from the racial pandemic. The qualitative study found Black men seeing themselves as positive, adaptive, and resourceful despite having less optimistic views about the United States overall.

Strengths are closely associated with resilience and have overt relevance for Black Americans participating in CBT. There has been a long-standing call for the strengths of Black Americans to be formally utilized in psychotherapy and research (White, 1980). In defining Black American strengths, the writings of texts addressing the strengths model (Rapp & Goscha, 2011) and perspective (Glicken, 2004) have been used. Strengths represent both the individual and collective, actual and potential positive resources that Black Americans bring to the psychotherapeutic process to achieve treatment goals and personal aspirations. These strengths may reside within the individual Black client, their family, community, history, and culture. A general precept of the Strengths principle is that all Black American clients have strengths regardless of any individual or collective disparities or socioeconomic disadvantages which may exist, and the strengths of Black American clients can be mobilized to aid in achieving constructive change. As seen in behavioral and social science research, Black American strengths are varied and powerful indicators of potential well-being. Kelly (2019) has identified Black cultural strengths that include social supports, spiritual beliefs, organized religion, and a positive racial identify. These factors may act as buffers against anti-Black racial stressors. Johnson and Carter (2020) validated a statistical model showing: communalism, a central and internalized racial identity, culturally based spirituality, socialization, and coping skills, were empirically associated with overall positive psychosocial outcomes. Another statistical model showed that Black families which were close and adaptable had decreased levels of individual stress and to a lesser extent spirituality was also empirically linked to decreased stress (Pollock et al., 2015). Qualitative research, examining Black men's coping with the racial pandemic, has found that culturally oriented spiritual, technological, appraisal/cognitive, and relational coping were deemed important coping mechanisms or strengths to be used against anti-Black racial injustice (Gregory Jr. & Tucker Edmonds, 2023). A statistical model by Opara and associates (2022) demonstrated a substantive and positive link between Black female youths' psychological empowerment and their ethnic identity. In summary, there is empirically supported evidence for various sources of strength in Black American culture and individuals.

4.2.1.1 Primary Function(s) of Principal 1: Cognitive-Behavioral Clinician

Within the context of CBT, the *Resilience and Strengths of Black Americans* principle calls for cognitive-behavioral clinicians to collaboratively and systematically identify and use the resilience and strengths of Black American clients to accomplish their treatment goals and personal aspirations. Theory and research have identified a number of converging Black American resilience and strengths factors: positive racial identity, spirituality, social support, autonomous and culturally informed coping skills for anti-Black racial stressors, and a collective Black conscious to fight anti-Black social injustice (Gregory Jr. & Tucker Edmonds, 2023; Johnson & Carter, 2020; Kelly, 2019; Opara et al., 2022; Pollock et al., 2015; Turner et al., 2022). Once resilience and strength factors are collaboratively identified, these factors could serve as evidence against internalized racism-oriented and other maladaptive anti-Black thoughts or beliefs (Hays, 2009; Steele, 2020). Beyond cognitive restructuring, clinicians could also use the identified resilience and strength factors to affirm and validate Black American clients, thereby building and sustaining therapeutic rapport and client self-efficacy. The aforementioned resilience and strengths factors are prominent in behavioral and social science. However, these factors will certainly vary in type, amount, and readiness to employ, according to each unique Black American client, their family, and their community. For further relevant discussion, see principle 9 on the *Uniqueness of Each Black Individual*.

4.2.2 *Principle 2: Empathy for Black Traumatic Events and Stressors*

Interpersonal empathy has been defined as the clinician's deliberate and communicated understanding of the client's experience (Ho, 2023). In psychotherapy, empathy has long been considered a minimally necessary component of therapeutic change (Rogers, 1957). Researchers have argued that empathy or other common factors are the prime determinants of psychotherapeutic progress (Messer & Wampold, 2002) and meta-analytic research has validated the importance of empathy in predicting psychotherapeutic outcomes (Elliott et al., 2018). Similarly, research has also underscored the importance of using empathy regarding Black culturally traumatic events, stressors (Aymer, 2016; Gregory Jr. & Tucker Edmonds, 2023), and discrimination (Gregory Jr., 2019). Empathy and other therapeutic rapport issues have traditionally been considered a principle for CBT (Beck, 2021). However, the strong history of empathy in psychotherapy has not always translated to Black trauma and race-based stressors (Tummala-Narra, 2020). Meta-analytic research has shown that denying structural racism was moderately linked to anti-Blackness (Yi et al., 2022). Therefore, given the importance of empathy as espoused by traditional CBT principles and research, cognitive-behavioral clinicians working with Black American clients improve the likelihood of a sound therapeutic rapport when empathy is clearly conveyed. The importance of conveying empathy to Black American clients is amplified as it pertains to issues of cultural trauma and race-based stressors. Empathy should be embodied in the cognitive-behavioral clinician's verbal and nonverbal communications, case conceptualizations, diagnostic considerations, and clinical documentation regarding Black American clients.

4.2.2.1 Primary Function(s) of Principal 2: Cognitive-Behavioral Clinician

The implications of empathy for Black traumatic events and stressors appear relatively straightforward. This principle is manifested in verbal and nonverbal communicative behaviors. These communicative behaviors convey an accurate and authentic understanding of Black American clients' perceptions and impacts of Black traumatic events and the structural forces which perpetuate them. The effective and consistent use of empathy should not detract from the effective use of cognitive restructuring and aspects of collaborative empiricism (see principle 6, *Evaluating Thoughts and Beliefs*, for further elaboration). While the presence and quality of empathy can often be measured in the cognitive-behavioral clinician's clinical encounters or experiences with the Black American client, empathy is also profoundly seen in how the cognitive-behavioral clinician chooses to conceptualize, diagnose, and clinically document the client's case. Cognitive-behavioral case conceptualizations for Black American clients should include clinically relevant structural factors that may substantively impact Black American clients' beliefs, thoughts, and behaviors (see Chap. 5 for further discussion). Considerations of how structural factors can influence Black American client's thoughts, behaviors, and health disparities require empathy. It is this prerequisite empathy that allows cognitive-behavioral clinicians to begin to understand how the broader American structures more accurately account for psychosocial functioning and other factors that intersect cognitive-behavioral treatment with Black Americans.

4.2.3 Principle 3: Structural Racism—Influences on Presenting Problems, Rapport, and Therapy

Very closely related to empathy is the third principle, *Structural Racism—Influences on Presenting Problems, Rapport, and Therapy*. For clarification, principle two speaks to a fundamental attribute of empathy that is required of the cognitive-behavioral clinician who is working with Black American clients who are impacted by structural inequity. However, the third principle addresses how structural factors impact Black Americans and how these structural factors are addressed in CBT. Chapter 2 outlined the roles US laws, policies, history, and different social systems have in creating and sustaining various biopsychosocial and economic disparities in Black Americans. The third principle calls for cognitive-behavioral clinicians to recognize and meaningfully account for these structural inequities in clinical practice. This principle calls for CBT clinicians to think critically about structural racism and develop therapeutic rapport, case conceptualizations, and treatment plans that mitigate or counter its clinical impact. Structural racism can lead to Black Americans being distrustful of the psychotherapeutic healthcare system (Gregory Jr. & Clary, 2022). On an interpersonal level, structural racism can contribute to the adoption of stereotypical or racist views of clinicians regarding Black American clients in psychotherapy (del Mar Fariña & O'Neill, 2022). These stereotypical, manifest or latent beliefs of clinicians can impede rapport building and effective cognitive-behavioral intervention with Black American clients.

4.2.3.1 Primary Function(s) of Principal 3: Cognitive-Behavioral Clinician

Depending on the Black American client who is engaged in CBT, the implementation of Principle 3 could vary a great deal. During the initial assessment, cognitive-behavioral clinicians should explore if and/or the extent to which structural racism may negatively impact the client's presenting problem. This exploration of structural factors can include closed and/or open-ended probing questions and/or the use of psychometric scales that quantify such aggravating structural factors. The Cultural Trauma Scale's (CuTS) *America and Its Justice System: Cognitive-Emotional Reponses* subscale is an excellent example of a psychometric measure that quantifies Black American perceptions of structural racism (Gregory Jr. & Tucker Edmonds, 2024a, 2024b). A copy of the 27 and 22 item versions of the CuTS are located in Appendices C and D, respectively. The initial and ongoing psychosocial assessments should inform the preliminary and evolving cognitive-behavioral case conceptualization of the Black American client, respectively. If structural factors are identified as being meaningful contributors to the presenting problem and/or the development of beliefs, these issues should be specified in the cognitive-behavioral case formulation. As indicated in CBT (Beck, 2021), the Black American client should also review and approve the case formulation. Beyond the client's psychosocial assessment, the cognitive-behavioral clinician must also be engaged in activities to raise their own awareness and circumvent the impacts of structural racism and implicit bias. These clinician-initiated activities include engaging in supervision and consultation regarding the provision of CBT with Black American clients and seeking client feedback regarding their perceptions of the therapy and the therapeutic relationship. These suggestions are only a starting point and not an exhaustive list of the ways in which anti-Black structural racism can be circumvented in the CBT process.

4.2.4 Principle 4: Problem-Solving

The fourth principle focuses on the necessity of *Problem-Solving*, as a clinical intervention with Black Americans who cope with mental illness and various forms of social injustice. Problem-solving, as an intervention with Black Americans, is justified in part by the reality of social inequity and its psychological implications. Some distressing experiences, situations, and emotions are due to an accurate appraisal of life circumstances, rather than a flawed perception of events. Cognitive-behavioral therapy includes the identification, testing, and modification of distorted thoughts (Beck, 2021). However, as is acknowledged in CBT (Leahy, 1996), sometimes clients' thoughts are true. In addition to the detrimental psychosocial consequences of racism and discrimination, Chap. 2 identified a history of structural factors which continue to contribute to Black disparities in finances, incarceration, health, and other social factors. Problem-solving is important given its utility for developing potential solutions to daily race-based stressors. The *Problem-Solving* principle in CBT with Black Americans can be understood using the framework of D'Zurilla & Nezu' (1999) relationalproblem-solving model. In this model, stress is explained via the interactive nature of distressing life events (major and routine stressors), emotional responses (positive and negative), and problem-solving coping (a process used to decrease stress). Black Americans encounter both major and daily anti-Black stressors (Stressful Life Events). The effects of these stressful events are mediated via culturally specific appraisals of the anti-Black stressors, coping resources, and use of coping strategies (Emotional Stress Responses). The problem-solving model or adaptations thereof can be used to aid in the mitigation of race-based stressors (Lewis-Coles & Constantine, 2006; Polanco-Roman et al., 2016).

4.2.4.1 Primary Function(s) of Principle 4: Cognitive-Behavioral Clinician

There are several cognitive-behavioral clinician oriented implications for the *Problem-Solving* principle. First is the acknowledgment that anti-Black discrimination and structural racism exists and are directly linked to psychological suffering and the exacerbation of psychiatric conditions experienced by Black Americans. As indicated in *Principle Two*, empathy for these race-based stressors is essential. While cognitive reconstruction has an important role in CBT with Black Americans (see Principle 6), problem-solving is a fundamental intervention that is used to address those situations that are rooted in structural and interpersonal racism and not explained by errors in appraisal. When addressing race-based problems in psychotherapy, Black Americans should be guided in using the problem-solving model (D'Zurilla & Nezu, 1999), to (1) Define the problem, (2) Identify possible solutions, (3) Evaluate the relative pros and cons of possible solutions, and (4) Implement and measure the effectiveness of the solution(s). As indicated, the problem-solving intervention should be done in a manner that is harmonious with the other CBT principles for Black Americans. In addition to resolving real-world, anti-Black race-based problems, the latent benefit of using problem-solving is to increase self-efficacy regarding the Black American's perceived ability to effectively respond to race-based stressors.

4.2.5 Principle 5: Policy Change

In addition to micro-level phenomena such as childhood experiences, beliefs, thoughts, and emotions encompassing Black American mental illness and psychological suffering, macro factors also substantively contribute to Black American mental illness and impede or enhance recovery (see Chap. 2). Principle 3, *Structural Racism—Influences on Presenting Problems, Rapport, and Therapy*, provided the racialized structural context of CBT with Black Americans and demonstrated the ways in which laws, policies, institutions, and various social systems directly or indirectly contribute to long-standing Black American disparities. These micro-level problems may become the primary reason for mental health treatment (for example, trauma stemming from racialized anti-Black violence) or may exacerbate pre-existing psychiatric diagnoses (worsening anxiety or depression due to racial discrimination). However, policy can also be a primary determinant of advances in social justice for Black Americans and consequently improved psychosocial functioning. Macro or upstream factors consistently contribute to or aggravate mental illness in Black Americans. Therefore, given the potential for policy to improve Black American mental health, the focus of *Principle Five* is *Policy Change*. In this principle, the term policy is inclusive of changes in laws, regulations, state statues, and federal legislation, which could be instrumental in improving Black American mental health, recovery, and overall psychosocial functioning.

4.2.5.1 Primary Function(s) of Principal 5: Cognitive-Behavioral Clinician

The primary function of the *Policy Change* principle, is the cognitive-behavioral clinician's understanding of and engagement in upstream-oriented activities to improve micro-level functioning for Black American clients with mental illness and addiction. Depending on the cognitive-behavioral clinician's discipline, training, professional skill set, and work setting, various forms of policy change efforts may be initiated. These activities could include necessary case management activities. For example, referring Black clients to access resources that are necessary to address the practical needs of an individual who is disproportionately exposed to various health disparities. Other policy-oriented efforts cognitive-behavioral clinicians can engage in to address Black American disparities include case and class advocacy, policy evaluation, policy advocacy, and policy development. These and other forms of policy change may be used by cognitive-behavioral clinicians given their exposure to Black American clients who may benefit from upstream/macro policy change that substantially aids in their psychosocial functioning. Arguably, the helping profession most readily available to engage in policy change to counter structural racism and improve Black American mental health would be social workers. The social work profession's emphasis on social justice, policy, and marginalized populations (National Association of Social Workers, 2023) makes it an obvious profession for engaging in some of the policy change efforts that are discussed in this principle. Professions such as nursing, psychiatry, psychology, and others also have unique attributes that may amplify policy change efforts used to advocate for Black American equity and mental health.

4.2.6 Principle 6: Evaluating Thoughts and Beliefs

4.2.6.1 The Utility of the Cognitive Model

The cognitive model (Beck, 1976) has provided a basic framework that allows cognitive restructuring to examine and replace irrational beliefs related to numerous Diagnostic Statistical Manual (DSM) psychiatric disorders (American Psychiatric Association, 2022). Diagnostic-specific cognitive models and manualized cognitive restructuring methods for addressing irrational beliefs pertaining to disorders of substance use (Beck et al., 1993; Wenzel et al., 2012), anxiety (Beck et al., 1985; Norton, 2012), depression (Beck et al., 1979), personality (Beck et al., 2015), psychosis (Beck et al., 2009), and others exist. As discussed in Chap. 1, although the literature is relatively scant, Black American clients can certainly benefit from these cognitive interventions as demonstrated in various meta-analyses (Gregory Jr., 2016, 2019; Montgomery et al., 2017). Cognitive restructuring methods with Black Americans may become more complex when maladaptive irrational beliefs specific to various diagnostic categories intersect with structural racism, discrimination, trauma, and/or varying degrees of internalized racism.

4.2.6.2 Black Maladaptive Beliefs and Their Structural Antecedents

The unique importance of cognitive restructuring with Black American clients is the best demonstrated via research, which has identified maladaptive beliefs and thoughts associated with discrimination, trauma, internalized, and structural racism. As indicated in principle 3 (*Structural Racism—Influences on Presenting Problems, Rapport, and Therapy*), Black-oriented maladaptive beliefs all have their origins in structural and racial disparities. See Chap. 6, section *Anti-Black Structural Injustice: Consequent Cognitive Distortions and Consequences*, for more on Black maladaptive beliefs stemming from structural racism. For example, the Strong Black Woman schema includes depression-oriented beliefs pertaining to limited self-expression and altruism (Beauboeuf-Lafontant, 2008). The Strong Black Woman schema has been shown to be empirically associated with problematic perfectionism, decreased self-compassion, and decreased use of coping (Liao et al., 2020). The strong Black woman schema stems from structural and racial disparities (Godbolt et al., 2022; Liao et al., 2020). More information regarding the Strong Black Woman Schema and cognitive restructuring is provided in Chap. 8. Based on an elaboration of Pyke's (2010) internalized racism definition, internalized anti-Black racism is the Black individual's adoption of negative, Black-denigrating beliefs about themselves and/or their Black culture. Internalized anti-Black racism is also rooted in structural racism (Speight, 2007). Research with Black American men has resulted in the Tripartite Model of Black Male Police Fear (Gregory Jr. & Tucker Edmonds, 2023, 2024a, 2024b). As it pertains to police violence, the model specifies Black men's fear for themselves, their families, and their families' fear for them. The construct of Tripartite Model of Black Male Police Fear was also validated in two independent psychometric analyses with Black Males (Gregory Jr. & Tucker Edmonds, 2024a, 2024b). This model is important not only due to the emotional, physiologic, and psychological consequences of police-related chronic fear (Miller & Vittrup, 2020), but also because of the distrust that associated with other structures (Gregory Jr. et al., in press; Gregory Jr. & Clary, 2022). For example, if a Black man experiences various forms of structural racism, the Black man's negative beliefs about those racist structures could be imputed onto systems such as mental healthcare, which could potentially be helpful to the Black man. The behavioral consequence of the belief that mental health systems are malicious could be the avoidance of mental healthcare, a reluctance to trust the providers, or reluctance to be fully invested in the process (Bauer et al., 2023). These potential negative beliefs could also pertain to Black men's perception that the provider is unable to relate to the Black client.

4.2.6.3 Cognitive Restructuring with Black Americans: Barriers to Implementation

The systematic and collaborative evaluation of thoughts and beliefs is a characteristic trait of CBT (Beck, 2021) and is substantially important when using CBT with Black Americans. Yet research has shown that clinicians find validation as having more utility than cognitive restructuring methods when working with Black clients (Ezawa & Strunk, 2022). Ezawa and Strunk concluded that clinicians were more likely to rate validation as being more appropriate than cognitive restructuring because the clinicians were concerned with minimizing or displaying a lack of belief regarding the Black clients' experiences. Cognitive restructuring, to the extent that the case conceptualization and/or clinical circumstances call for it, is as important as validation in the context of CBT. The second principle in this chapter focuses on *Empathy*, which includes various forms of validation. Both cognitive restructuring and validation are synergistic in CBT (Beck et al., 1979). Black American clients, addressing psychiatric diagnostic and/or racial issues (discrimination, trauma, internalized racism) can and should be validated, and this validation does not need to occur at the expense of cognitive restructuring methods. A defining feature of CBT is the labeling, examining, and modifying of cognitive distortions. If cognitive restructuring is not being substantively employed in CBT with Black Americans in a manner that is responsive to the cognitive-behavioral case conceptualization, a legitimate question arises as to why CBT is even being used with the Black American client?

4.2.6.4 Primary Function(s) of Principal 6: Cognitive-Behavioral Clinician

The primary functions of principle six (*Evaluating Thoughts and Beliefs*), involve cognitive restructuring in a collaborative, empathetic (principle 2), and structurally informed (principle 3) manner, which makes constructive use of each Black client's individual and collective resilience and strength (principle 1). The Black client should comprehend the cognitive model, so the proposed mechanisms, by which cognitive restructuring interventions achieve their effect can be understood. First, identify and explain the major components of the cognitive model (Beck, 2021): thoughts/beliefs about situations can lead to changes in emotions and behavior. Discuss the mediating influence of thoughts/beliefs on behaviors and emotions (Ellis, 1994). Individualized, culturally relevant scenarios that illustrate the cognitive model can be presented. Examples used to illustrate the cognitive model may come from the situations identified in the Black client's initial assessment, case conceptualization, and current or past culturally relevant situations that the client has shared. Questions for and feedback to the Black client can be used to collaboratively illustrate how the cognitive model explains negative and positive changes in emotion and behavior. It must be stated that each Black individual is unique (see principle 9, *Uniqueness of Each Black Individual*). So culturally relevant situations used to elucidate the cognitive model will vary a great deal from one Black client to another. Once the cognitive model is understood and a framework for classifying thoughts and beliefs has been discussed, core Socratic questions are used in CBT to create positive emotional and behavioral change (Beck, 2021; Beck et al., 1979; Leahy, 1996). These core Socratic questions typically evoke responses that facilitate the client's examination of the:

- Extent to which thoughts/beliefs are and are not supported by objective evidence.
- Advantages and disadvantages of thoughts/beliefs.
- Practicality or plausibility of thoughts/beliefs.
- Universality of thoughts/beliefs (does the thought apply equally to others?)
- Alternative possibilities for the way in which a situation is interpreted.
- Potential actions that can be taken to address a situation.

These different types of Socratic questions can typically be distinguished by their emphasis on empiricism (Evidence), functionality (advantages and disadvantages), philosophy (practicality and plausibility), and action-oriented strategies (Bishop, 2001). The individual and collective resilience and strengths of each Black client vary among Black clients (see principle 9, *Uniqueness of Each Black Individual*). Socratic questions may be used to mobilize a Black client's idiosyncratic strengths and resilience (Principle 1: *Resilience and Strength of Black Americans*) by asking the client questions that embody or explore intrapersonal and collective strengths realized through overcoming adversity, actual or potential strengths in relationships, community connections or resources, positive Black identity, and spiritual beliefs or scriptures (Gregory Jr. & Tucker Edmonds, 2023; Johnson & Carter, 2020; Kelly, 2019; Opara et al., 2022; Pollock et al., 2015; Turner et al., 2022). These Socratic questions that target a Black client's strengths and resilience may be useful in countering maladaptive thoughts/beliefs stemming from specific psychiatric disorders and associated discrimination, trauma, and/or internalized racism.

4.2.7 Principle 7: Critical Evaluation of Clinical and Other Relevant Research

Research plays a crucial role in the provision and funding of psychotherapeutic services. Several terms have been used to explain the empirical base for interventions in psychotherapy. *Empirically Supported Psychological Therapies* were characterized by psychotherapeutic interventions which were manualized and demonstrated superiority in RCTs or other research designs (Chambless & Hollon, 1998). A more nuanced definition, *Evidence-Based Practice*, involves the use of research, the professional opinion of the clinician, and the needs and desires of the client to guide psychotherapeutic intervention (Drisko & Grady, 2015). Drisko and Grady's definition of evidence-based practice shares similarities with what others have defined as *Evidence-Informed* practice (Miles & Loughlin, 2011). How do these issues relate to principle 7, *Critical Evaluation of Clinical and other Relevant Research*? Cognitive-behavioral therapy and evidence-based practice are quite congruent with one another (Hunsley & Elliott, 2015). However, evidence-based practices (Joyce, 2019) and CBT (Huey Jr et al., 2023) have legitimately been critiqued for their lack of emphasis on external validity. Relative to internal validity (methodological rigor that allows for causal conclusions), external validity (generalizability of results) has been underemphasized in clinical, behavioral research. This was Stanley Sue's critique of psychological science in 1999. The lack of external validity for Black Americans, in CBT research evaluating clinical outcomes creates a challenge that clinicians must reconcile in psychotherapeutic work with Black Americans. As emphasized in principle 3 (*Structural Racism—Influences on Presenting Problems, Rapport, and Therapy*), some Black clients may have distrust for the healthcare system and psychotherapy given long-standing structural racism that is often denied or not acknowledged. When working as a clinician in a community mental health center, the author vividly recalled a Black male client, who was court-ordered to treatment, asking me if he (referring to other Black individuals) was included in any of these studies that the author used to partially explain why he was recommending CBT. The lack of Black representation in samples of RCTs evaluating CBT for various psychiatric disorders may contribute to cynicism and distrust among Black clients. For these reasons, cognitive-behavioral clinicians should view RCTs, meta-analyses, and other clinical research critically, not only to determine the methodological features (internal validity), but also the extent to which Black clients are included in the studies (external validity).

4.2.7.1 Primary Function(s) of Principal 7: Cognitive-Behavioral Clinician

Given the available and limited research that exists on CBT with Black Americans, clinicians working with Black Americans will have to first ask if Black participants were included in the study. However, this alone is not enough. Black Americans are not simply Black; they are Black male, Black female, Black with a Hispanic ethnicity, Black youth, and Black in addition to a number of other intersectional demographic qualities. Therefore, cognitive-behavioral clinicians need to critically evaluate research not only for Black Americans, but depending on the client they are working with, other intersectional identities may be of particular importance. This emphasis on intersectionality also speaks to the importance of principle 9, addressing the *Uniqueness of Each Black Individual.* A critical evaluation of Black relevant CBT research may also require some increased understanding of research methodology and statistical analysis. For example, when there are not enough RCTs to conduct a thorough meta-analysis of psychotherapeutic outcomes for Black participants, sometimes moderator analyses are used to help overcome this limitation. Moderator analyses in meta-analytic studies may include statistical techniques such as meta-regression or subgroup analyses (Borenstein et al., 2021). In meta-regression, the percentage of Black individuals in the studies will be used to predict the overall treatment outcome effect size. Subgroup analyses make statistical comparisons between groups to determine if the effect sizes from each subgroup are significantly different.

The primary function of principle 7 is not to encourage master level clinicians to obtain more statistical training. Instead, the primary function of principle 7 is to simply suggest the need for critical evaluation of clinical research as it relates to Black Americans. Clinicians can use this critical evaluation to aid in honest and transparent communications, about the evidence-base of CBT with Black American clients. An instance was described above, where a Black male client asked the author if he (referencing other Black individuals) was included in any of the CBT research the author discussed. The author's response included an honest, conversational, jargon-free description of the evidence-base for CBT with Black Americans and its limitations. The author discussed with the client, culturally adapted CBT, disorder specific meta-analyses limited to Black Americans, and research with Black Americans that is still needed. Within the context of evidence-based practice (Drisko & Grady, 2015), the Black American client was provided with empirical information, which could be integrated with other factors, to aid him in determining if he wanted to participate in CBT with the author.

4.2.8 Principle 8: Truth and Transparency

The principle of *Truth and Transparency* may seem redundant given Rogers's (1957) necessary conditions for therapeutic change and CBT's long-standing emphasis on genuineness (Beck et al., 1979). However, truth and transparency are of particular importance given the potential detrimental implications on therapeutic rapport, should a Black client perceive the clinician as dishonest or untrustworthy. The negative consequences of perceived clinician dishonesty and untrustworthiness are amplified by historical structural racism (see Chap. 2), inherent professional power differences between Black clients and their clinicians (Edge & Lemetyinen, 2019), and disparities in Black client engagement and retention in psychotherapy (Joiner et al., 2022). The negative synergy created by simultaneous, long-standing anti-Black racism and perceived clinician dishonesty can be disastrous for therapeutic rapport. A perceived lack of clinician truth or transparency can converge with historical anti-black racism and result in Black clients dropping out of treatment prematurely and/or developing despairing views of psychotherapy that may later inhibit engagement or retention. While maladaptive beliefs of all types may appear to be an excellent fit for CBT, Black clients must first be engaged in treatment before any maladaptive beliefs about therapy can be challenged or substantively disconfirmed by experience.

4.2.8.1 Primary Function(s) of Principal 8: Cognitive-Behavioral Clinician

Beck and associates (1979) maintain that clinicians are to be honest with themselves and with their clients. Arguably, the most useful exercise of principle 8 is in proactively creating a therapeutic culture of truth and transparency. This culture of Truth and Transparency includes not only the clinician, but also clinical supervisors and agency policy. There are an infinite number of client and clinician characteristics, clinical situations, and contextual circumstances about which issues of truth and transparency may arise. Therefore, this book adopts no prescriptive stance regarding how issues of truth and transparency are to absolutely manifest themselves. Take, for example, a number of clinical issues which may complicate the application of this principle. These issues include, but are not at all limited to mandatory reporting due to suspected child abuse, the clinician's views of sensitive and culturally traumatic incidents, and the depth of the therapeutic rapport between the Black client and the clinician. Much of the work for the Truth and Transparency principle with Black clients in CBT is done before the clinician sees their first Black client. Truth and transparency in CBT with Black clients may be partially achieved by those clinicians who have meaningful, substantive, and healthy experiences and relationships with a diverse number of Black individuals, although this is not always possible. Clinical supervision that regularly addresses therapeutic rapport with Black Americans and healthy and productive professional relationships with Black colleagues may begin to build a foundation of Truth and Transparency with Black clients.

To reiterate, Beck et al. (1979) have described the importance of CBT clinician's honesty with themselves and their clients. Therefore, self-awareness of the clinician's own beliefs about Black American clients, the origin of these beliefs, and continued work to challenge and replace counterproductive beliefs that inhibit clinical work with Black clients, are of the utmost importance. The clinician's continued self-awareness of how their verbal and written communications with and about Black American clients reflect their own beliefs and values will also contribute to Truth and Transparency in clinical relationships with Black American clients. See principle 2, *Empathy for Black Traumatic Events and Stressors*, for additional discussion regarding verbal and written communications regarding Black American clients.

4.2.9 Principle 9: Uniqueness of Each Black Individual

Principle 9, *Uniqueness of Each Black Individual*, emphasizes the within-group diversity in Black America. Relative to hackneyed depictions of Black Americans as poor and universally dark skinned (Celious & Oyserman, 2001), the diversity of Black Americans is demonstrated in:

- Beliefs about a wide range of historical events and social problems.
- Educational attainment.
- Gendered experiences.
- Geographic location (rural, suburban, and urban).
- Hobbies and interests.
- Phenotype (skin color and other physical attributes).
- Political affiliations.
- Psychiatric diagnoses.
- Religious beliefs and practices.
- SES.
- Substance use history.
- Talents.
- Countless other attributes.

An exhaustive summary of Black American statistics regarding each of the aforementioned categories is beyond the scope of the book. The key point is, no matter how strong a statistic is regarding issues of Black American identity and psychosocial attributes, there is always the fact that the Black client receiving CBT does not belong to the stereotypical category to which the Black American may be frequently delegated. For example, Black Americans have had a strong Democratic political affiliation in the United States (Wamble et al., 2022), yet this does not guarantee that Black American receiving treatment in CBT will be liberal minded. There are a number of dangers associated with stereotypical categorizations of Black Americans. These negative consequences include but are not limited to damage to the development and/or maintenance of therapeutic rapport, inaccurate diagnoses and treatment plans, flawed cognitive-behavioral case conceptualizations, demoralization of Black American clients, cynicism, or distrust of the psychotherapeutic healthcare system.

The *Uniqueness of Each Black Individual*, must be contrasted with the attributes of structural racism. As outlined in Chap. 2, structural racism has evolved overtime in American Institutions and society to recreate and sustain inequities in Black American liberty and prevent the full enjoyment and protection of US constitutional rights. Based on the history of structural racism in America, there are frequently documented biopsychosocial Black American disparities. Without exception, these disparities, which stem from structural racism, do not undermine or compromise the diversity or heterogeneity that exist within Black Americans. For example, the War on Drugs was associated with frequent depictions of BLACK Americans experiencing negative consequences or being perpetrators of cocaine use and distribution (Alexander, 2010), this does not mean that all or most Black Americans struggle with or are particularly at risk for substance use disorders. Black Americans represent 13.6% of the US population (US Census Bureau, n.d.); however, 35% of people in jails were Black (BJS, 2022). This finding does not mean that Black individuals are prone to criminality.

4.2.9.1 Primary Function(s) of Principal 9: Cognitive-Behavioral Clinician

The *Uniqueness of Each Black Individual* principle recognizes the within group diversity among Black American clients and uses Black heterogeneity to inform work with Black clients. One of the primary functions of this principle is for the CBT clinician to do a thorough initial assessment and continue to provide substantive ongoing assessments of the Black client. Both the initial and ongoing assessments are used to allow cognitive-behavioral interventions to be uniquely tailored to the specific client's unique attributes and case conceptualization. In Chap. 6, Cognitive-Behavioral Interventions with Black Americans, examples of cognitive-behavioral interventions and their connections to Rodgerick's case conceptualization and initial and ongoing assessments are provided.

Given the actual and potential deleterious effects of disregarding the *Uniqueness of Each Black Individual*, it is important that each cognitive-behavioral therapist not impute characteristics of Black American clients based on race or stereotypical notions of race. Similar to the functions or principal 8, *Truth and Transparency*, cognitive-behavioral clinicians must first be honest with themselves regarding their own beliefs (Beck et al., 1979) about Black Americans and the origin of these beliefs. Once these beliefs are identified, continued self-monitoring and challenging the empirical evidence of such beliefs may be of benefit to clinicians who hold biased beliefs of Black clients. Tendencies to categorize Black Americans according to racialized stereotypes may also be addressed via professional supervision. There are circumstances where the cognitive-behavioral clinician's narrow view of Black Americans and/or Black culture will negatively influence the provision of services to Black Americans and become harmful. In such instances, the cessation of therapeutic services to the Black American client is appropriate, and reassignment to a clinician who does not hold harmful anti-Black beliefs is appropriate. Ideally, individuals providing CBT to Black Americans would see the within-group plurality and failure to do so would be caught early on in therapy and addressed before any harm to the therapeutic rapport and/or client occurs.

4.2.10 Principle 10: Social Support's Import

The tenth and final principle addresses the importance and utility of social support in CBT with Black Americans. The first principle, *Resilience and Strengths of Black Americans*, identified relationships as one factor that potentially contributes to Black fortitude against racial stressors and social injustice (Turner et al., 2022). There is substantial research that shows Black American social support is a buffer against racial discrimination and psychological distress (Benca-Bachman et al., 2020; Gregory Jr. & Tucker Edmonds, 2023; Jacob et al., 2023; Muruthi et al., 2023; Qin et al., 2020; Ramseur II et al., 2023; Salami et al., 2021; Steers et al., 2019; Williams, 2022), suicide risk factors (Khan et al., 2021; Reed et al., 2021), and substance use (Sartor & Black, 2021). Several of these studies have begun to evaluate the potential, empirical mechanisms by which social support may aid Black Americans in coping with racial discrimination and psychological distress.

4.2.10.1 Primary Function(s) of Principal 10: Cognitive-Behavioral Clinician

The primary function of principle ten, *Social Support's Import*, is to highlight and guide cognitive-behavioral therapists in aiding Black American clients in engaging and sustaining social support networks that may be beneficial for racial discrimination, various forms of psychological distress, and other stressors. The exact type and amounts of social support will depend on the Black American client's preferences, relevant information from assessment, the ongoing case conceptualization, and clinically relevant research. Meta-analytic research has provided some evidence that perceived social support may be more important than actual social support (Park et al., 2014). For some Black Americans, there may be several extant and adaptive sources of social support. Yet, there may be thoughts and beliefs that create a barrier to accessing those adaptive sources of support. In these cases, the identification and subsequent challenging of thoughts may be a necessary precursor to engaging beneficial social support networks. See principle 6, *Evaluating Thoughts and Beliefs*, for more additional information regarding cognitive restructuring with Black Americans. In other cases, barriers created by distance, racial homogeneity (environments were access to other Black individuals is limited), or lack of financial resources may complicate or impede access to adaptive social support networks. For these barriers, principle 4, *Problem-Solving*, should be used to co-create and evaluate potential solutions to overcome these obstacles.

4.3 Interdependence of the Ten Cognitive-Behavioral Principles for Black Americans

The ten principles are interdependent and were conceptualized to be harmonious with one another, while incorporating clinically relevant Black American research findings. Due to the interdependence of the principles, when appropriate, each principle references other principles that may aid clinicians in enhancing CBT with Black Americans. For example, principle 2: *Empathy for Black Traumatic Events and Stressors* or principle 8: *Truth and Transparency* can easily be considered as applying to all sessions with Black Americans. In other circumstances, depending on the Black American client's diagnosis, case conceptualization, preferences, and the cognitive-behavioral clinician's guidance there may be times when some principles may be used more prominently than others. Take, for example, a session with a Black American client that involves a depressive disorder. It may not be until later sessions that issues of evaluating the thoughts or beliefs (principle 6: *Evaluating Thoughts and Beliefs*) become more relevant.

4.4 Potential Candidates for the Cognitive-Behavioral RESPPECTUS Principles

In accordance with Principle 9, Uniqueness of Each Black Individual, not all Black individuals in America are the same. Therefore, the utility of the cognitive-behavioral principles for Black Americans are best viewed from a continuous rather than a categorical perspective. The principles were written to have the broadest beneficial impact among all Black Americans. Given the focus on Black strengths, Black persons with substantial internalized racism may not immediately appreciate the utility of the principles. The author anticipates that the cognitive-behavioral RESPPECTUS principles may have the most utility for Black Americans with a positive Black identity, Black individuals for whom structural racism has hindered engagement or retention in psychotherapy, Black individuals whom present with a clinical issue or DSM diagnosis that is integrally related to structural racism (for example, cultural trauma), and Black individuals who believe that the therapist's background (constant factors that the therapist has no ability to change) precludes a positive therapeutic rapport or working relationship.

4.5 Cognitive-Behavioral RESPPECTUS Principles for Black Americans: Summary

The present chapter discussed the ten cognitive-behavioral RESPPECTUS principles for Black Americans and their primary function for the cognitive-behavioral clinician. The ten cognitive-behavioral principles for Black Americans were:

Principle 1: Resilience and strengths of Black Americans.
Principle 2: Empathy for Black traumatic events and stressors.
Principle 3: Structural racism–influences on presenting problems, rapport, and therapy.
Principle 4: Problem-solving.
Principle 5: Policy change.
Principle 6: Evaluating thoughts and beliefs.
Principle 7: Critical evaluation of clinical and other relevant research.
Principle 8: Truth and transparency.
Principle 9: Uniqueness of each Black individual.
Principle 10: Social support's import.

The principles have theoretical and empirical support. The principles are collectively referred to by their acronym RESPPECTUS. The interdependent nature of the principles and some considerations regarding Black Americans who may be optimal candidates for the principles are discussed.

Chapter 5 discusses the application of the CBT principles for Black Americans, pertaining to cognitive-behavioral case conceptualization. Frequently used scales and important constructs relevant to cognitive-behavioral treatment of Black Americans are identified and discussed. The Cultural Trauma Scale (CuTS; Gregory Jr. & Tucker Edmonds, 2024a, 2024b) is presented as a scale which has been psychometrically validated in Black American men and measures constructs which are relevant for CBT and structural racism. An illustration of a cognitive-behavioral case conceptualization, using the RESPPECTUS principles with the case of Rodgerick is provided in the next chapter.

References

Alexander, M. (2010). *The new Jim Crow: Mass incarceration in the ages of colorblindness*. The New Press.

American Psychiatric Association. (2022). *Diagnostic and statistical manual of mental disorders* (5th ed., text rev.). https://doi.org/10.1176/appi.books.9780890425787.

Aymer, S. R. (2016). "I can't breathe": A case study—Helping Black men cope with race-related trauma stemming from police killing and brutality. *Journal of Human Behavior in the Social Environment, 26*(3/4), 367–376. https://doi.org/10.1080/10911359.2015.1132828

Bauer, A. G., Christensen, K., Bowe-Thompson, C., Lister, S., Aduloju-Ajijola, N., & Berkley-Patton, J. (2020). "We are our own counselor": Resilience, risk behaviors, and mental health service utilization among young African American men. *Behavioral Medicine, 46*(3/4), 278–289. https://doi.org/10.1080/08964289.2020.1729087

Bauer, A. G., Williams, J., Hambrick, E., Rempfer, M., Bennett, K., Christensen, K., & Berkley-Patton, J. Y. (2023). Mental health attitudes, norms, beliefs, and experiences with care among young Black men: A theory of planned behavior assessment. *Psychological Trauma Theory Research Practice and Policy* https://doi.org/10.1037/tra0001462.supp (Supplemental).

Beauboeuf-Lafontant, T. (2008). Listening past the lies that make us sick: A voice-centered analysis of strength and depression among Black women. *Qualitative Sociology, 31*(4), 391–406. https://doi.org/10.1007/s11133-008-9113-1

Beck, A. T. (1976). *Cognitive therapy and the emotional disorders*. Meridian.

Beck, J. S. (2021). *Cognitive behavior therapy: Basics and beyond* (3rd ed.). Guilford Press.

Beck, A. T., Davis, D. D., & Freeman, A. (Eds.). (2015). *Cognitive therapy of personality disorders* (3rd ed.). Guilford Press.

Beck, A. T., Emery, G., & Greenberg, R. L. (1985). *Anxiety disorders and phobias: A cognitive perspective*. Basic Books.

Beck, A. T., Rector, N. A., Stolar, N., & Grant, P. (2009). *Schizophrenia: Cognitive theory, research, and therapy*. Guilford Press.

Beck, A. T., Rush, A. J., Shaw, B. F., & Emery, G. (1979). *Cognitive therapy of depression*. Guilford Press.

Beck, A. T., Wright, F. D., Newman, C. F., & Liese, B. S. (1993). *Cognitive therapy of substance abuse*. Guilford Press.

Benca-Bachman, C. E., Najera, D. D., Whitfield, K. E., Taylor, J. L., Thorpe, R. J., & Palmer, R. H. C. (2020). Quality and quantity of social support show differential associations with stress and depression in African Americans. *The American Journal of Geriatric Psychiatry, 28*(6), 597–605. https://doi.org/10.1016/j.jagp.2020.02.004

Bishop, F. M. (2001). *Managing addictions: Cognitive, emotive, and behavioral techniques*. Jason Aronson.

Borenstein, M., Hedges, L. V., Higgins, J. P. T., & Rothstein, H. R. (2021). *Introduction to meta-analysis* (2nd ed.). John Wiley & Sons.

Bronfenbrenner, U. (1977). Toward an experimental ecology of human development. *American Psychologist, 32*(7), 513–531. https://doi.org/10.1037/0003-066X.32.7.513

Bureau of Justice Statistics. (2022, December 20). *U.S. jail population increased while prison population decreased in 2021*. https://bjs.ojp.gov/sites/g/files/xyckuh236/files/media/document/p21st_ji21st_prB.pdf

Carson, E. A. (2020). *Prisoners in 2019*. Bureau of Justice Statistics. https://bjs.ojp.gov/content/pub/pdf/p19.pdf

Celious, A., & Oyserman, D. (2001). Race from the inside: An emerging heterogeneous race model. *Journal of Social Issues, 57*(1), 149–165. https://doi.org/10.1111/0022-4537.00206

Chambless, D. L., & Hollon, S. D. (1998). Defining empirically supported therapies. *Journal of Consulting and Clinical Psychology, 66*(1), 7–18. https://doi.org/10.1037/0022-006X.66.1.7

D'Zurilla, J. J., & Nezu, A. M. (1999). *Problem-solving therapy: A social competence approach to clinical intervention* (2nd ed.). Springer Publications Company.

del Mar Fariña, M., & O'Neill, P. (2022). The structural clinical model: Disrupting oppression in clinical social work through an integrative practice approach. *Clinical Social Work Journal*. https://doi.org/10.1007/s10615-022-00841-3

Drisko, J., & Grady, M. (2015). Evidence-based practice in social work: A contemporary perspective. *Clinical Social Work Journal, 43*(3), 274–282. https://doi.org/10.1007/s10615-015-0548-z

Edge, D., & Lemetyinen, H. (2019). Psychology across cultures: Challenges and opportunities. *Psychology and Psychotherapy: Theory, Research and Practice, 92*(2), 261–276. https://doi.org/10.1111/papt.12229

Elliott, R., Bohart, A. C., Watson, J. C., & Murphy, D. (2018). Therapist empathy and client outcome: An updated meta-analysis. *Psychotherapy (Chicago, Ill.), 55*(4), 399–410. https://doi.org/10.1037/pst0000175

Ellis, A. (1994). *Reason and emotion in psychotherapy: A comprehensive method of treating human disturbances (revised and updated)*. Carol Publishing Group.

Ezawa, I. D., & Strunk, D. R. (2022). Working with Black vs. White patients: An experimental test of therapist decision-making in cognitive behavioral therapy for depression. *Cognitive Behaviour Therapy, 51*(3), 229–242. https://doi.org/10.1080/16506073.2021.1970799

Glicken, M. D. (2004). *Using the strengths perspective in social work practice*. Ally and Bacon.

Godbolt, D., Opara, I., & Amutah-Onukagha, N. (2022). Strong Black women: Linking stereotypes, stress, and overeating among a sample of Black female college students. *Journal of Black Studies, 53*(6), 609–634. https://doi.org/10.1177/00219347221087453

Gregory, V. L., Jr. (2016). Cognitive-behavioral therapy for depressive symptoms in persons of African descent: A meta-analysis. *Journal of Social Service Research, 42*(1), 113–129. https://doi.org/10.1080/01488376.2015.1084973

Gregory, V. L., Jr. (2019). Cognitive-behavioral therapy for anxious symptoms in persons of African descent: A meta-analysis. *Journal of Social Service Research, 45*(1), 87–101. https://doi.org/10.1080/01488376.2018.1479344

Gregory, V. L., Jr., & Clary, K. L. (2022). Addressing anti-Black racism: The roles of social work. *Smith College Studies In Social Work, 92*(1), 1–27. https://doi.org/10.1080/00377317.2021.2008287

Gregory, V. L., Jr., Miller, B. L., & Lipsey, A. (in press). Black men, structural racism, cultural barriers: Structural equation model with cognitive-behavioral implications. *The Counseling Psychologist*.

Gregory, V. L., Jr., & Tucker Edmonds, J. L. (2023). The racial pandemic experienced by Black American men: Cognitive-behavioral and structural implications. *American Journal of Orthopsychiatry, 93*(1), 1–16. https://doi.org/10.1037/ort0000651

Gregory, V. L., Jr., & Tucker Edmonds, J. L. (2024a). Cultural trauma scale: Psychometric evaluation of Black men's beliefs, emotions, and coping. *Psychological Trauma Theory Research Practice and Policy, 16*(8), 1329–1337. https://doi.org/10.1037/tra0001607

Gregory, V. L., Jr., & Tucker Edmonds, J. L. (2024b). Cultural trauma scale (CuTS): Parsimonious principal component analysis, independent Black American male sample. *Journal of Aggression, Maltreatment & Trauma, 33*(3), 369–386. https://doi.org/10.1080/10926771.2023.2256741

Gurpinar-Morgan, A., Murray, C., & Beck, A. (2014). Ethnicity and the therapeutic relationship: Views of young people accessing cognitive behavioural therapy. *Mental Health, Religion and Culture, 17*(7), 714–725. https://doi.org/10.1080/13674676.2014.903388

Hays, P. A. (2009). Integrating evidence-based practice, cognitive–behavior therapy, and multicultural therapy: Ten steps for culturally competent practice. *Professional Psychology: Research and Practice, 40*(4), 354–360. https://doi.org/10.1037/a0016250

Ho, C. (2023). Process of interpersonal empathy: A proposed framework of empathy competence in psychotherapies. *Person-Centered & Experiential Psychotherapies, 23*(1), 39–53. https://doi.org/10.1080/14779757.2023.2174446

Huey, S. J., Jr., Park, A. L., Galán, C. A., & Wang, C. X. (2023). Culturally responsive cognitive behavioral therapy for ethnically diverse populations. *Annual Review of Clinical Psychology, 19*, 51–78. https://doi.org/10.1146/annurev-clinpsy-080921-072750

Hunsley, J., & Elliott, K. (2015). Implementing an evidence-based approach to cognitive-behavioral assessment. In G. P. Brown & D. A. Clark (Eds.), *Assessment in cognitive therapy* (pp. 121–145). The Guilford Press.

Jacob, G., Faber, S. C., Faber, N., Bartlett, A., Ouimet, A. J., & Williams, M. T. (2023). A systematic review of Black people coping with racism: Approaches, analysis, and empowerment. *Perspectives on Psychological Science, 18*(2), 392–415. https://doi.org/10.1177/17456916221100509

Johnson, V. E., & Carter, R. T. (2020). Black cultural strengths and psychosocial well-being: An empirical analysis with Black American adults. *Journal of Black Psychology, 46*(1), 55–89. https://doi-org.proxy.ulib.uits.iu.edu/10.1177/0095798419889752

Joiner, T. E., Robison, M., Robertson, L., Keel, P., Daurio, A. M., Mehra, L. M., & Millender, E. (2022). Ethnoracial status, intersectionality with gender, and psychotherapy utilization, retention, and outcomes. *Journal of Consulting and Clinical Psychology, 90*(10), 837–849. https://doi.org/10.1037/ccp0000726

Joyce, K. E. (2019). The key role of representativeness in evidence-based education. *Educational Research and Evaluation, 25*(1–2), 43–62. https://doi.org/10.1080/13803611.2019.1617989

Judge, A. S., Downing, K. F., Nembhard, W. N., Oster, M. E., & Farr, S. L. (2023). Racial and ethnic disparities in socio-economic status, access to care, and healthcare utilisation among children with heart conditions, national survey of children's health 2016–2019. *Cardiology in the Young, 1–9*. https://doi.org/10.1017/S1047951122004097

Kahneman, D. (2011). *Thinking, fast and slow*. Farrar, Straus, and Giroux.

Kelly, S. (2019). Cognitive behavior therapy with African Americans. In G. Y. Iwamasa & P. A. Hays (Eds.), *Culturally responsive cognitive behavior therapy: Practice and supervision., 2nd ed* (pp. 105–128). American Psychological Association. https://doi.org/10.1037/0000119-005

Khan, H., Zhang, S., Gutowski, E., Jessani, S. N., & Kaslow, N. J. (2021). Does social support moderate between depression and suicidal ideation in low-income African Americans? *The American Journal of Orthopsychiatry, 91*(5), 617–625. https://doi.org/10.1037/ort0000561

Kiesewetter, J., & Huber, J. (2021). A primer of an in-depth resilience status for German medical graduates: Results of a cross-sectional survey on the status quo of resilience among graduates of human medicine in Bavaria, Germany—A necessary step in building an emotionally equipped healthcare work-force. *BMC Medical Education, 21*(1), 573. https://doi.org/10.1186/s12909-021-02933-z

Knight, Z. G. (2013). Black client, White therapist: Working with race in psychoanalytic psychotherapy in South Africa. *International Journal of Psychoanalysis, 94*(1), 17–31. https://doi.org/10.1111/1745-8315.12034

Leahy, R. (1996). *Cognitive therapy: Basic principles and applications*. Jason Aronson.

Lewis-Coles, M. E. L., & Constantine, M. G. (2006). Racism-related stress, Africultural coping, and religious problem-solving among African Americans. *Cultural Diversity & Ethnic Minority Psychology, 12*(3), 433–443. https://doi.org/10.1037/1099-9809.12.3.433

Liao, K. Y.-H., Wei, M., & Yin, M. (2020). The misunderstood schema of the strong Black woman: Exploring its mental health consequences and coping responses among African American women. *Psychology of Women Quarterly, 44*(1), 84–104. https://doi.org/10.1177/0361684319883198

Messer, S. B., & Wampold, B. E. (2002). Let's face facts: Common factors are more potent than specific therapy ingredients. *Clinical Psychology: Science and Practice, 9*(1), 21–25. https://doi.org/10.1093/clipsy.9.1.21

Miles, A., & Loughlin, M. (2011). Models in the balance: Evidence-based medicine versus evidence-informed individualized care. *Journal of Evaluation in Clinical Practice, 17*(4), 531–536. https://doi.org/10.1111/j.1365-2753.2011.01713.x

Miller, C., & Vittrup, B. (2020). The indirect effects of police racial bias on African American families. *Journal of Family Issues, 41*(10), 1699–1722. https://doi.org/10.1177/0192513X20929068

Montgomery, L., Robinson, C., Seaman, E. L., & Haeny, A. M. (2017). A scoping review and meta-analysis of psychosocial and pharmacological treatments for cannabis and tobacco use among African Americans. *Psychology of Addictive Behaviors, 31*(8), 922–943. https://doi.org/10.1037/adb0000326

Muruthi, J. R., Muruthi, B. A., Thompson Cañas, R. E., Romero, L., Taiwo, A., & Ehlinger, P. P. (2023). Daily discrimination, church support, personal mastery, and psychological distress in Black people in the United States. *Ethnicity & Health, 28*(4), 503–521. https://doi.org/10.1080/13557858.2022.207848

National Association of Social Workers (NASW). (2023). *Code of ethics of the national association of social workers*. Author.

Norton, P. J. (2012). *Group cognitive-behavioral therapy of anxiety: A transdiagnostic treatment manual*. Guilford Press.

Opara, I., Lardier, D. T., Jr., Garcia-Reid, P., & Reid, R. J. (2022). Measuring intrapersonal psychological empowerment and ethnic identity: Highlighting strengths of urban Black girls. *Youth & Society, 54*(4), 573–592. https://doi.org/10.1177/0044118X20970226

Park, M., Cuijpers, P., Straten, A., & Reynolds, C. (2014). The effects of psychotherapy for adult depression on social support: A meta-analysis. *Cognitive Therapy and Research, 38*(6), 600–611. https://doi.org/10.1007/s10608-014-9630-z

Polanco-Roman, L., Danies, A., & Anglin, D. M. (2016). Racial discrimination as race-based trauma, coping strategies, and dissociative symptoms among emerging adults. *Psychological Trauma Theory Research Practice and Policy, 8*(5), 609–617. https://doi.org/10.1037/tra0000125

Pollock, E. D., Kazman, J. B., & Deuster, P. (2015). Family functioning and stress in African American families: A strength-based approach. *Journal of Black Psychology, 41*(2), 144–169. https://doi.org/10.1177/0095798413520451

Pyke, K. D. (2010). What is internalized racial oppression and why don't we study it? Acknowledging racism's hidden injuries. *Sociological Perspectives, 53*(4), 551–572. https://doi.org/10.1525/sop.2010.53.4.551

Qin, W., Nguyen, A. W., Mouzon, D. M., Hamler, T. C., & Wang, F. (2020). Social support, everyday discrimination, and depressive symptoms among older African Americans: A longitudinal study. *Innovation in Aging, 4*(5), igaa032. https://doi.org/10.1093/geroni/igaa032

Ramseur, K., II, Cattaneo, L. B., Stori, S., & Adams, L. (2023). Black men need friends: Social support moderates the connection between gendered racism and psychological distress. *Psychology of Men & Masculinities*. https://doi.org/10.1037/men0000449

Rapp, C. A., & Goscha, R. J. (2011). *A recovery-oriented approach to mental health services* (3rd ed.). Oxford University Press.

Reed, D. D., Stoeffler, S. W., & Joseph, R. (2021). Suicide, race, and social work: A systematic review of protective factors among African Americans. *Journal of Evidence-Based Social Work (2019), 18*(4), 379–393. https://doi.org/10.1080/26408066.2020.1857317

Rogers, C. R. (1957). The necessary and sufficient conditions of therapeutic personality change. *Journal of Consulting Psychology, 21*(2), 95–103. https://doi.org/10.1037/h0045357

Rogers, T. N., Rogers, C. R., VanSant-Webb, E., Gu, L. Y., Yan, B., & Qeadan, F. (2020). Racial disparities in COVID-19 mortality among essential workers in the United States. *World Medical & Health Policy, 12*(3), 311–327. https://doi.org/10.1002/wmh3.358

Salami, T., Lawson, E., & Metzger, I. W. (2021). The impact of microaggressions on Black college students worry about their future employment: The moderating role of social support and academic achievement. *Cultural Diversity and Ethnic Minority Psychology, 27*(2), 245–255. https://doi.org/10.1037/cdp0000340

Sartor, C. E., & Black, A. C. (2021). Profiles of psychosocial risk and protective factors and their associations with alcohol use and regular smoking in Black adults. *Journal of Racial and Ethnic Health Disparities, 8*(1), 60–68. https://doi.org/10.1007/s40615-020-00754-2

Speight, S. L. (2007). Internalized racism: One more piece of the puzzle. *The Counseling Psychologist, 35*(1), 126–134. https://doi.org/10.1177/0011000006295119

Steele, J. M. (2020). A CBT approach to internalized racism among African Americans. *International Journal for the Advancement of Counselling, 42*(3), 217–233. https://doi.org/10.1007/s10447-020-09402-0

Steers, M.-L. N., Chen, T.-A., Neisler, J., Obasi, E. M., McNeill, L. H., & Reitzel, L. R. (2019). The buffering effect of social support on the relationship between discrimination and psychological distress among church-going African-American adults. *Behaviour Research and Therapy, 115*, 121–128. https://doi.org/10.1016/j.brat.2018.10.008

Sue, S. (1999). Science, ethnicity, and bias: Where have we gone wrong? *American Psychologist, 54*(12), 1070–1077. https://doi.org/10.1037/0003-066X.54.12.1070

Tummala-Narra, P. (2020). Racial trauma and dissociated worlds within psychotherapy: A discussion of racial difference, rupture, and repair: A view from the couch and back. *Psychoanalytic Dialogues, 30*(6), 732–741. https://doi.org/10.1080/10481885.2020.1829437

Turner, E. A., Harrell, S. P., & Bryant-Davis, T. (2022). Black love, activism, and community (BLAC): The BLAC model of healing and resilience. *Journal of Black Psychology, 48*(3/4), 547–568. https://doi.org/10.1177/00957984211018364

United States Census Bureau. (n.d.). *Quickfacts United States*. https://www.census.gov/quickfacts/fact/table/US/RHI225221

Wamble, J. J., Laird, C. N., McConnaughy, C. M., & White, I. K. (2022). We are one: The social maintenance of Black democratic party loyalty. *Journal of Politics, 84*(2), 682–697. https://doi.org/10.1086/716300

Wenzel, A., Liese, B. S., Beck, A. T., & Friedman-Wheeler, D. G. (2012). *Group cognitive therapy for addictions*. The Guilford Press.

White. J. L. (1980). Toward a Black psychology. In R. Jones (Ed.). (2004). *Black psychology* (2nd ed., pp. 5–12). Harper & Row.

Williams, E. K. (2022). Racial socialization and perceived social support for African American fathers in academia. *Family Relations: An Interdisciplinary Journal of Applied Family Studies, 71*(5), 1949–1972. https://doi.org/10.1111/fare.12796

Yi, J., Neville, H. A., Todd, N. R., & Mekawi, Y. (2022). Ignoring race and denying racism: A meta-analysis of the associations between colorblind racial ideology, anti-blackness, and other variables antithetical to racial justice. *Journal of Counseling Psychology, 70*(3), 258–275. https://doi.org/10.1037/cou0000618

Chapter 5
Cognitive-Behavioral Case Conceptualization with Black Americans

5.1 Cognitive-Behavioral Case Conceptualization

Cognitive-behavioral case conceptualization was previously defined in Chap. 3's discussion of implicit racism, in the *Cognitive-Behavioral Case Conceptualization* section. In this chapter, a definition of the cognitive-behavioral case conceptualization is briefly reiterated. Case conceptualizations provide a theoretical representation of the client's presenting issues, difficulties, and provide a foundation for the client's individually tailored treatment plan (Persons et al., 2001). The case conceptualization calls for the identification of maladaptive thoughts that may contribute to the Black client's emotions and behavior. Cognitive-behavioral case conceptualization requires clinically relevant information to be gathered from clients. Qualitative feedback from clients has utility not only for the cognitive-behavioral case conceptualization but also for the overall cognitive-behavioral process.

5.2 Qualitative Feedback from Black American Clients: Case Conceptualization, Therapy, and the CBT RESPPECTUS Principles

Open-ended questions or qualitative feedback provide a less precise way of summarizing Black American clients' thoughts about any number of events. Obtaining client feedback at the end of sessions has been recommended by Beck and Associates (1979). The qualitative, open-ended feedback obtained from clients at the end of each session can be used to help modify the ongoing cognitive-behavioral case conceptualization. Seeking qualitative feedback from Black American clients at the end of sessions can often provide thick descriptive details regarding the

V. L. Gregory, Jr., *Cognitive-Behavioral Therapy with Black Americans*,
https://doi.org/10.1007/978-3-032-01666-9_5

session, which may be of particular importance for the client and the clinician as they collaboratively address treatment goals. Requesting, seriously considering, and effectively using client feedback at the end of sessions is an excellent way to demonstrate principle 8, *Truth and Transparency* with Black Americans. The feedback from Black clients allows the Black clients to discuss any issues, questions, or misunderstandings that may potentially threaten the therapeutic rapport. This overt request for feedback embraces truth and transparency as it provides a routine time for Black American clients to voice any potential concerns or seek further clarification and understanding regarding the CBT session. Clinically relevant, case conceptualization information that may be derived from seeking client feedback includes potential insights that may be gleaned regarding the trust or distrust of the mental healthcare system. If the Black client feedback converges with structural factors and allows for a more engaging conversation regarding how structural factors influence the treatment process or treatment goals, then seeking such feedback may also embody principle 3, *Structural Racism—Influences on Presenting Problems, Rapport, and Therapy*. For non-Black clinicians, seeking and taking seriously Black client feedback may disconfirm some cynicism or distrust that the Black client may have for the therapist and/or the psychotherapeutic healthcare system. For Black clinicians, seeking client feedback may rebut some potential misgivings that Black clients may have for their race-concordant clinicians. For example, some race-concordant dyads (clinician and client), may involve the Black client believing that the Black therapist is overconfident in assuming they know what the client is experiencing based exclusively on their shared racial background (Gurpinar-Morgan et al., 2014). Seeking client feedback may help disconfirm this as well. The specific benefits of qualitative Black client feedback include the potential strengthening of the therapeutic rapport (Beck, 2021) via such feedback being requested and the clinician's response demonstrating empathy for the Black client (see principle 2, *Empathy for Black Traumatic Events and Stressors* principle).

5.3 Psychometric Scales

In addition to seeking qualitative, session-based feedback from Black clients, there is much clinical gain in case conceptualization that can be experienced from the use of psychometrically validated clinical measures. Psychometrically validated scales can be used in cognitive-behavioral case conceptualization to help identify specific cognitive distortions, areas of strength and resilience, presenting problems, as well as quantify clinically relevant Black constructs. The psychometrically validated scales of Black constructs, should be used in conjunction with other clinical forms of data collection, including but not limited to psychosocial assessments and interviews.

5.3.1 Symptoms and Quality of Life

There are numerous scales which measure symptoms and quality of life. For example, the Patient Health Questionnaire-9 (PHQ-9; Kroenke et al., 2001), Generalized Anxiety Disorder-7 (GAD-7; Spitzer et al., 2006), Satisfaction with Life Scale (SWLS; Diener et al., 1985), the Rosenberg Self-Esteem Scale (RSES; Rosenberg, 1989), and countless other scales which may be used depending on the Black client's diagnosis and treatment goals.

5.3.2 Strengths

Similarly, several scales exist which measure client strengths. These strength-oriented scales include but are certainly not limited to the recovery-oriented Adult Needs and Strengths Assessment (ANSA; Lyons & Walton, 2007) scale and the Client Assessment of Strengths, Interests and Goals (CASIG; Wallace et al., 2001). Both of the ANSA (Walton & Kim, 2018) and the strength-bases scales have been psychometrically validated. The psychometric evaluation of the ANSA contained a Black sample (13.1%) that closely approximated the US population of Black Americans. Evidence of cross-cultural validity for symptom or strength-based scales with Black samples will use psychometric methods such as factor analyses, measurement and structural invariance analyses (Bryne, 2016), item response theory, and/or Cronbach's Alpha (Cronbach, 1951), among others.

5.4 Black Constructs: Psychometrically Validated Scales

The term Black constructs, represents those latent variables that are germane to Black American strengths, culturally specific clinical outcomes, and social challenges. Scales measuring Black-relevant constructs can be used in conjunction with the aforementioned clinical measures that are unrelated to the client's race. The concurrent use of such scales aids in the assessment and monitoring of both symptomatic (intrapersonal) and race-based psychosocial constructs (intrapersonal and environmental) which are pertinent to treatment. As is true with other psychometric measures (Nunnally & Bernstein, 1994), scales quantifying Black constructs also have the advantages of objective measurement, communication, and efficiency. The measurement of Black constructs, using psychometrically validated scales, allows for the development of the case conceptualization and the assessment of target outcomes over the course of the cognitive-behavioral intervention.

Table 5.1 provides a descriptive overview of psychometrically validated scales which measure Black constructs. The table provides a quick overview of the scale's names, constructs measured by each of the scale's subscales, type of factor analysis

Table 5.1 Black constructs: psychometrically validated scales

Scales	Author(s)	Black subscale construct categories							N	Sample	Factor analysis		Validity		Cronbach's alpha subscale range
		Coping	Discrimination/ racism/stress	Internalized racism	Interpersonal	Resilience/ strengths	Structural Factors	Trauma/ symptoms			EFA[a]	CFA	Construct[b]	Criterion	
AARS-M	Briggs et al. (2022)				X	X			161	100% Blk, M		X	X		0.74–0.89
AARS-W	↓				X	X			117	100% Blk, F		X	X		0.50–0.82
BMES	Bowleg et al. (2016)		X			X			578	100% Blk, M	X	X	X		0.71–0.84
CuTS	Gregory & Tucker Edmonds (2024a)[c]	X				X	X	X	240	100% Blk, M	X		X		0.61–0.88
CuTS (SV)	Gregory & Tucker Edmonds (2024b)[c]	X				X	X	X	150	100% Blk, M	X		X		0.64–0.84
HTS	Williams-Washington and Mills (2018)		X		X	X		X	342	100% Blk, M&F	X		X		0.91[c]
IROS	Bailey et al. (2017)			X					468	100% Blk, M&F	X	X	X		0.77–0.83
IRRS	Utsey and Ponterotto (1996)		X				X		302	100% Blk, M&F	X		X		0.79–0.87
IRRS-B	Utsey (1999)		X				X		239	100% Blk, M&F		X	X		0.69–0.78
RBTSSS	Carter et al. (2013)							X	320	32.8% Blk, M&F	X		X		0.66–0.96

↓	Carter and Muchow (2017)							↓	1.1 k	47.9% Blk, M&F		X	X	X	0.73–0.90
↓	Carter et al. (2018)							↓	527	100% Blk, M&F		X	X	X	0.84–0.92
↓	Pieterse et al. (2023)							↓	148	52.7%, Blk, M&F			X		0.76–0.95
REMS	Nadal (2011)		X		X				443	18% Blk, M&F	X		X		0.78–0.87
RRCS	Forsyth and Carter (2014)	X							307	100% Blk, M&F	X		X		0.70–0.90
RTS	Williams et al. (2022)							X	339	51% Blk, M&F	X		X	X	0.93–0.95
↓	↓							↓	326	35% Blk, M&F		X	X	X	0.90–0.95
TSDS	Williams et al. (2018)		X					X	123	100%[d] Blk, M&F	X		X	X	0.94

AARS-M African American Respect Scale-Men, *AARS-W* African American Respect Scale-Women, B-Brief version, *Blk* Black, BMES—Black Male Experiences Scale, *CFA* Confirmatory Factor Analysis, *CuTS* Cultural Trauma Scale, *EFA* Exploratory Factor Analysis, *F* female, *HTS* Historical Trauma Scale, *IROS* Internalized Racial Oppression Scale, *IRRS-B* Index of Race-Related Stress Brief Version, *k* 1000, *M* male, *REMS* Racial and Ethnic Micro Aggressions Scale, *RBTSSS* Race-Based Traumatic Stress Symptom Scale, *RRCS* Racism Related Coping Scale, *RTS* Racial Trauma Scale, *TSDS* Trauma Symptoms of Discrimination Scale, *SV* short version

[a]Principal component analysis was considered an EFA for the purposes of summarizing the scales

[b]EFA, during initial psychometric evaluation, was considered evidence of construct validity; CFA, the a priori model, have a better fit to the data that competing models, is also considered evidence of construct validity (Worthington & Whittaker, 2006)

[c]There were four factors in this scale, the total scale Cronbach's alpha was reported

[d]This sample includes persons who are biracial and Black Americans

used to support the scales' factorial validity, evidence of other forms of validity, internal consistency reliability, the extent of Black representation in the sample, and references for readers to obtain more information about the scales. Scales presented in the table were selected due to their psychometric properties and their relevance to Black discrimination, trauma, and internalized racism. For each of the scales included in the table, the scales' constructs are classified according to Black: (1) Coping, (2) Discrimination/racism/racial stress, (3) Internalized racism, (4) Interpersonal factors (respect), (5) Resilience/strength, (6) Structural factors, and racialized trauma and symptoms. Interpersonal factors are distinguished from the other categories, because they include social issues which are not necessarily negative. Discrimination/racism/racial stress, given that the latter is always negative, and the former is not. Readers can use the table for a quick summary to aid in considering whether the scale may be appropriate for their Black American clients. The table is not exhaustive, and readers must use the appropriate sources to determine if and how they may be able to use the scales (copyright issues).

Additional scales, with relevance for Black Americans experiencing racism, discrimination, and trauma are provided in the systematic review conducted by Kirkinis and colleagues (2021) and available elsewhere in the behavioral science literature. The CuTS (Gregory & Tucker Edmonds, 2024a, 2024b, is provided in Appendices C and D. Readers must review the appropriate sources to determine the intellectual property issues associated with each scale.

5.4.1 Black Constructs: Case Conceptualization, Therapy, and the CBT RESPPECTUS Principles

As seen in Table 5.1, there are many psychometrically validated scales, measuring constructs of particular relevance to Black Americans. These scales have the potential to be clinically useful and aid in facilitating the cognitive-behavioral RESPPECTUS principles with Black American clients. When using psychometrically validated scales for case conceptualization and treatment purposes with Black Americans, the cognitive-behavioral clinician should be sure the scale has been validated in a Black sample that is representative of their client. The use of cross-culturally validated measures with Black clients embodies principle 7, *Critical Evaluation of Clinical and other Relevant Research,* and helps ensure that there is psychometric support for using the scale with the Black client. When using a scale with a Black client, the CBT clinician should know that the scale has evidence of validity and reliability for the Black client. In Table 5.1, measures which evaluate the specific strengths of Black Americas are identified and discussed. The first principle, may be quantified for Black men using the Resilience subscale of the Cultural Trauma Scale (CuTS; Gregory & Tucker Edmonds, 2024a, 2024b), the Family subscale of the African American Respect Scale for men (AARS-M; Briggs et al., 2022), or the Positives: Black Men subscale of the Black Men Experiences Scale

(BMES). The AARS for women (Briggs et al., 2022) also identifies factors with direct relation to strengths and resilience. Identifying and using Black client strengths embodies the first principle of *Resilience and Strength of Black Americans*. These scales, which assess strength and/or resilience can be used to help identify positive Black client attributes for the case conceptualization. Beyond the case conceptualization, the content of these resilience and strengths-based subscales may be used to identify evidence that is contrary to maladaptive thoughts and beliefs or to create self-talk that fosters more adaptive thoughts and beliefs (principle 6, *Evaluating Thoughts and Beliefs*). The number of items on these subscales ranges between three and five items, making them brief and efficient measures. These scales, tapping the constructs of Black resilience and strength, are also important due to their potential to quantify positive clinically or statistically significant changes that may not be observed in scales that are purely deficit or symptom-based (Shedler, 2010).

As stated in Chap. 2, anti-Black structural racism creates or contributes to negative psychosocial consequences, including worsening mental health (Cavalhieri et al., 2023), trauma (Gregory & Tucker Edmonds, 2023), and internalized racism (Mouzon & McLean, 2017). The measurement of trauma for the initial assessment, cognitive-behavioral case conceptualization, and ongoing treatment is supported by principle 2, *Empathy for Black Traumatic Events and Stressors* principle. In cognitive-behavioral case conceptualization, measures of trauma could be used to help identify relevant issues for the problem list. Many of the scales identified in Table 5.1 provide various quantifications of trauma that are disproportionately experienced in the Black community, for example, trauma pertaining to police interactions (Edwards et al., 2019; Gregory & Tucker Edmonds, 2024a, 2024b). As it pertains to other forms of cultural trauma (CuTS; Gregory & Tucker Edmonds, 2024a, 2024b), the Historical Trauma Scale (HTS; Williams-Washington & Mills, 2018), the Race-Based Traumatic Stress Symptom Scale (RBTSSS; Carter et al., 2013, 2018; Pieterse et al., 2023), and the Trauma Symptoms of Discrimination Scale (TSDS; Williams et al., 2018) have been psychometrically validated with samples who were exclusively Black. Beyond providing decreased error in measurement, these scales may also be used to open important discussions about Black Trauma and its impact on mental illness and addiction. Black trauma is rooted in structural racism. Structural racism creates functional consequences (mass incarceration, for example) that contribute to Black disparities in employment, education, wealth, and other aspects of American society (Alexander, 2010). Discussions of trauma and its consequences will and should lead to a search for practical solutions. It is the search for practical solutions which necessitate problem-solving approaches (principle 4, *Problem-Solving*) to address and correct socioeconomic disparities. There were far fewer scales measuring internalized racism with Black individuals. The Internalized Racial Oppression Scale (IROS, Bailey et al., 2017) is one such scale that has been validated with an exclusively Black sample.

In addition to scales that measure Black trauma, there were two scales, with subscales that measured the constructs of structural racism. The CuTS's Beliefs about America and its Justice System and Tripartite Police Fear (Gregory & Tucker

Edmonds, 2024a, 2024b) subscales and the Index of Race-Related Stress, Institutional Racism subscale (IRRS; Utsey, 1999; IRRS-Utsey & Ponterotto, 1996) were among the few scales that measured structural racism. Principle 3 addresses *Structural Racism—Influences on Presenting Problems, Rapport, and Therapy*. High scores on these subscales, quantifying structural racism, provide the CBT therapist with a quantitative view of the Black client's perspective on American institutions, police fear, and the broader world.

The a priori use of scales measuring Black constructs may be tailored according to the clinical needs of the Black clients served by the agency, the agency's mission, and the Black clients' unique clinical circumstances. Readers are recommended to use the appropriate sources to determine if and how they may be able to use the scales (copyright issues). Two versions of the CuTS (Gregory & Tucker Edmonds, 2024a, 2024b) are located in the appendixes C and D of the present text.

5.5 Cognitive-Behavioral Case Conceptualization with Black American Clients: The Role of Structures

Following an initial assessment, scales measuring Black constructs may potentially aid in the case formulation of Black American clients and their presenting problems. Case formulation is a person-specific theory that provides an explanation for a client's symptoms and creates the foundation for a treatment plan to direct therapy (Persons et al., 2001). As stated by Persons (1989), irrational beliefs are major contributors to clients' maladaptive thoughts, emotions, and behaviors. Persons (1989) has described how the interdependent nature of thoughts, emotions, and behavior explains some of the mechanisms by which various evidence-based CBTs work. In addition to these psychological phenomena, Persons (1989) states that environmental issues also have an influential role in stimulating irrational beliefs and consequent psychological symptoms. In the model proposed by Persons (1989), the psychological phenomena are mutually interactive. However, the same cannot be said for various environmental or structural factors that may trigger irrational beliefs in Black Americans. While cognitive and behavioral interventions may help facilitate healing from the psychosocial sequalae of structural racism (Gregory & Tucker Edmonds, 2023), healing or psychosocial intervention alone will not nullify or deter the upstream causes of anti-Black racism (Corley & Young, 2018). Principles 3 (*Structural Racism—Influences on Presenting Problems, Rapport, and Therapy*) and 5 (*Policy Change*) provide context and clinical guidance for these circumstances. The traditional case formulation identification of relevant cognitive structures, symptoms, interventions, diagnoses, etcetera (Persons, 2008) aids in addressing micro-level symptoms and personal goals for psychotherapy. Cognitive-behavioral case formulation with Black Americans seeks to acknowledge the role of structural factors in contributing to Black American mental health problems and broader racial disparities. This structural component of the case formulation lays the groundwork for problem-solving (principle four) to address structural issues and their micro-level consequences.

5.6 Biopsychosocial Assessment

The biopsychosocial model, proposed by Engel (1977), takes into account psychological, sociological, biological, and cultural components when considering the origins and treatment of disease/disorders. Engle also discussed the similarities and synchrony between the biopsychosocial assessment and the general system theory discussed by Bertalanffy (1969). The primary tenets of Engle's biopsychosocial model are also compatible with the general systems theory (Nichols & Davis, 2017) that was discussed in Chap. 1. The biopsychosocial model is a more wholistic approach to assessment of Black American clients and is necessary to begin identifying and addressing the various micro, mezzo, and structural factors which will ultimately influence the implementation of CBT with many Black American clients. Below is an example of a biopsychosocial assessment and case conceptualization. The case of Rodgerick is used as a narrative example.

5.7 Cognitive-Behavioral Biopsychosocial Assessment: Black Male Exemplar with Rodgerick

The case of Rodgerick is a hypothetical vignette that is loosely based on the author's years of experience working with Black clients using CBT. Many of the Black clients with whom the author worked experienced various forms of Black trauma and different mental illness and substance use diagnoses, which are aggravated by or stemmed from structural racism. Rodgerick is a 19-year-old, Black American, male client who has been diagnosed with a DSM-5 (American Psychiatric Association, 2022) Generalized Anxiety Disorder (300.02). Aspects of Rodgerick's psychosocial assessment are provided below.

5.7.1 Presenting Concerns

Rodgerick reports that his coming to treatment was based on overall fear that he has had since high school. Rodgerick states that this fear has increased greatly since being in college. Specific areas of great concern to Rodgerick include his grades for college, dating, money, and concerns about what others think of him. Rodgerick states that his worry has made him physically ill and has decreased his ability to relax and enjoy aspects of his life that should otherwise be enjoyable. Rodgerick reports that he is anxious about everyday situations, big events, and long-term goals for his future.

5.7.2 Physical/Medical

Rodgerick reports having high blood pressure and a vitamin D deficiency. Rodgerick states that his high blood pressure has not been diagnosed or treated; however, he reports taking a vitamin D supplement. The report of a vitamin D deficiency has been confirmed by information released by Rodgerick's primary care physician. Rodgerick attributes his high blood pressure to his stress, his eating fast food routinely, and a lack of physical activity due to his primary focus being on studying and his grades.

5.7.3 Current Living Situation

Rodgerick currently lives with his mother. Rodgerick spends most of his time taking courses at a nearby college and working part-time. Both Rodgerick and his mother live in a middle-class, predominantly White neighborhood.

5.7.4 Family of Origin

Rodgerick reports having a tenuous and estranged relationship with his father, who lives just miles away from Rodgerick and Rodgerick's mother. Rodgerick has two older siblings (no longer living with him and his mother) and reports having healthy and supportive relationships with them. Rodgerick describes his upbringing as very strict yet loving. Rodgerick reports having an overall good relationship with his mother. He describes his mother as being overprotective during his childhood and states she still struggles with letting him "grow up." Rodgerick states that his mother has always been particularly fearful regarding Rodgerick being the victim of street and/or police violence.

5.7.5 Extended Family

As it pertains to extended family, Rodgerick reports that he has several aunts and one uncle who are supportive and available when Rodgerick reaches out to them. Rodgerick stated that he looked up to his uncle because his uncle was a mechanical engineer and a leader in his family. Rodgerick reports being close to his extended family. Rodgerick reports having some cousins (his uncle's children) who are more like brothers than cousins. Rodgerick reports that he is close in age to his uncle's children.

5.7.6 *Abuse/Neglect*

Rodgerick denies having ever been physically or sexually abused. However, Rodgerick does report that he believes his relationship with his father is emotionally abusive and sometimes thinks that his father "plays games with me" because of his father's sometimes strained relationship with Rodgerick's mother. Rodgerick reports that he has typically always had supervision as a child; however, there were a few times as a child when both of his parents worked, and he would spend the first several hours after school alone.

5.7.7 *Education*

Rodgerick is a sophomore in college, pursuing a bachelor's degree in secondary education. Rodgerick reports his current GPA is 3.15/4.00. Rodgerick attends and commutes to a campus located in the city in which he lives. The college is predominantly White; however, some pockets of racial diversity are present, per Rodgerick. Rodgerick reports believing that several of his professors have low expectations for his ability to excel in his coursework and grade him unfairly. Rodgerick reports that he attributes this to his being a Black male and the racial and gender bias of his professors. Prior to taking tests, Rodgerick states that his anxiety usually helps him perform better on the tests. Rodgerick reports worrying the most about his grades, between the time of assignment/test submission and receipt of his grade.

5.7.8 *Social*

Rodgerick states that he has many acquaintances, yet few friends. He reports that most of the friends he had have since gone out of state to college or are focused primarily on working. Rodgerick reports finding it difficult to relate to the majority of students at his college. Rodgerick reports that he is particularly concerned about dating, as there are very few Black women in his college courses. Rodgerick reports that these concerns are compounded when he thinks about the "fact that" even if he did meet another Black woman in one of his courses, the odds that she would be single or even like him are unlikely. Rodgerick reports typically being involved in school and other social settings where he is the only or one of very few Black individuals. Rodgerick reports believing that he will probably never have an active or rewarding dating life. Rodgerick states that he's unlikely to have a serious dating life because he has so little contact with other Black women at his school, and his social circle is not that big with regard to other Black people his age. Rodgerick recounted negative experiences with being alone in high school and feeling left out as he was not able to find someone of the same race (which he preferred) to go to the prom with. Yet, Rodgerick reports that over time he has become accustomed to "not only surviving but thriving" in places and social situations where he is racially isolated. However, Rodgerick states that he has continued to struggle as it pertains to finding Black female peers to develop relationships with.

5.7.9 Religion/Spirituality

Rodgerick reports being a Christian and states that his family has been involved with the church since he was a child. Rodgerick states that the family's frequency of church attendance has fluctuated over the years. Rodgerick reports knowing some Biblical scriptures, routinely engaging in prayer, and still having faith in God despite his not currently being an active member of any church.

5.7.10 Employment

Rodgerick is employed part-time at a grocery store. Rodgerick states that he, for the most part, is liked and accepted by his employers and the customers. However, Rodgerick reports that there are occasions when he believes customers are rude and states that his being Black certainly does not increase the likelihood that customers will be kind. Rodgerick reports that he sometimes does not have transportation home, and on occasion, people will yell things while driving by him in their cars. Despite this, Rodgerick reports not feeling physically threatened when he must walk home from work.

5.7.11 Criminal History

Rodgerick reports that he has never been arrested before, yet states that he has had more than one interactions with the police. Rodgerick states that his police interactions involve various issues in his neighborhood, with the police being called and a general sense that the police are not to be trusted.

5.7.12 *Prior Mental Health Treatment*

Rodgerick states, this is his first time in mental health treatment. Rodgerick reports that he initially believed that a mental health treatment center would be more appropriate for "other people" and "not someone like me."

5.7.13 *Anxiety*

Rodgerick reports that he has discussed his anxiety with his primary care physician, and he and the physician discussed the possibility of Rodgerick being prescribed Prozac (Fluoxetine). Rodgerick states that this discussion made him feel even more anxious, and he decided he would handle it on his own. Until the symptoms became too much and catalyzed his coming to the outpatient clinic. Rodgerick reports that he thinks a lot about bad stuff happening and reports that this "drives him crazy." Ironically, Rodgerick also report believing that his frequent thinking about problems and worrying helps keep him from experiencing negative outcomes. Rodgerick self-reports that his thinking is negative. Rodgerick states that he often doubts his own ability to effectively address his anxiety and control his worrying.

5.7.13.1 Generalized Anxiety Disorder-7 (GAD-7; Spitzer et al., 2006)

At intake, Rodgerick completed the GAD-7 and scored a 17 out of 21, which is considered severe anxiety. Rodgerick reports that his symptoms have made his life "Very difficult."

5.7.14 *Depression*

Rodgerick reports some depression. Yet Rodgerick reports that his main concern is his anxiety and states that depression is less of an issue. During his interview for the biopsychosocial assessment, Rodgerick did verbally acknowledge some aspects of the depressive cognitive triad (Beck et al., 1979). Rodgerick reports that, given the limitations on functioning caused by his anxiety, he does view himself as "not good enough," less competent, and more fearful than others his age. Rodgerick also states that he views his future negatively because his thoughts inevitably lead to the worst-case scenario.

5.7.14.1 Patient Health Questionnaire-9 (PHQ-9; Kroenke et al., 2001)

Rodgerick's completion of the PHQ-9 showed his depression to be at the upper threshold of a mild level, with Rodgerick scoring a 9 out of 27. Rodgerick reported that the depressive symptoms have made his life "Somewhat difficult."

5.7.15 *Cultural Trauma*

As it pertained to racial discrimination and/or racial stressors, Rodgerick had previously discussed racism and or discrimination in the context of his education and interactions with law enforcement. Due to the current and historical cultural traumatic events suffered by the Black community as a whole and individuals within the community, cultural trauma was formerly assessed, in consideration of ways in which cultural trauma may need to be represented in Rodgerick's case conceptualization and treatment plan. Rodgerick was given the 27-item Cultural Trauma Scale (CuTS; Gregory & Tucker Edmonds, 2024a) to complete. The CuTS 27 (located in Appendix C, Gregory & Tucker Edmonds, 2024a) version allows an unaltered version of the scale to be used only for noncommercial educational and research purposes, by appropriately trained personnel, as long as the source is cited. As it pertains to forthcoming CBT, the CuTS was given to Rodgerick to quantify various aspects of cultural trauma which may influence his treatment for GAD and to further facilitate discussion regarding his previous concerns about racial injustice and discrimination. It was also believed that empathic and non-judgmental discussion of issues pertaining to racism, social injustice, and discrimination may aid in building rapport with Rodgerick. This communicative expectation is embodied in principle 2, *Empathy for Black Traumatic Events and Stressors*.

5.7.15.1 America and Its Justice System: Cognitive-Emotional Responses—CuTS Subscale (Gregory & Tucker Edmonds, 2024a)

For the America and Its Justice System: Cognitive-Emotional Responses CuTS subscale, composite scores can range between 10 and 70, with higher scores indicating more distrust or cynicism for America and the criminal justice system. Rodgerick scored a 46/70, indicating a substantive degree of concern regarding social justice in America as it pertains to Black individuals. This quantified score was used to provide some context for Rodgerick's perception of anti-Black structural racism. In accordance with principle 3 (*Structural Racism—Influences on Presenting Problems, Rapport, and Therapy*), this also gives the cognitive-behavioral clinician additional insight as it pertains to the role and weight of structural racism in

Rodgerick's cognitive-behavioral case conceptualization. The America and Its Justice System: Cognitive-Emotional Responses subscale also has huge implications for principles 4 and 5, *Problem Solving* and *Policy Change*, respectively. The beliefs about America and its criminal justice system (items one through ten of the CuTS) are supported by a wide array of research and historical context that was outlined in Chap. 2 of the present text. Therefore, various upstream or structural factors substantively impact the psychosocial functioning and suffering of Black Americans. An appropriate response is not only how to cognitively, behaviorally, and emotionally respond to injustice, but also to recognize and address the structural factors that create and sustain various forms of Black trauma and socioeconomic disparity. The cognitive-behavioral clinician's approach to addressing upstream/structural factors regarding their Black clients will undoubtedly vary according to the clinician's professional training, skill set, state laws and legislative factors, licensure, professional supervision, continuing education, other professional, and idiosyncratic factors. At a bare minimum, the cognitive-behavioral clinician can acknowledge the structural factors which create and sustain various forms of social injustice and inequity within the United States.

5.7.15.2 Cognitive-Behavioral Coping Skills—CuTS Subscale (Gregory & Tucker Edmonds, 2024a)

The Cognitive-Behavioral Coping Skills subscale of the CuTS has 7 items, with a composite score range between 7 and 49. Higher scores are indicative of more CBT coping skills, which can be used to address anti-Black racism and discrimination. The Cognitive-Behavioral Coping Skills subscale can also be used to identify individual level strengths in coping, which may be used to inform the Black client's cognitive-behavioral case conceptualization. Despite Rodgerick's limited self-efficacy pertaining to coping with anxiety and aforementioned errors in thinking pertaining to anxiety and depression, Rodgerick scored a 42/49 on the Cognitive-Behavioral Coping Skills subscale. Specific items for which Rodgerick scored higher were discussed further to validate those coping skills as strengths and potential resources for addressing his anxiety symptoms. This subscale can potentially be used to underscore the first principle of *Resilience and Strength of Black Americans* by identifying potential coping skills or resources that Black clients may have access to or may currently be using.

As it pertains to Rodgerick's cognitive-behavioral case formulation, the Cognitive-Behavioral Coping Skills subscale of the CuTS can be used to apply principle 6: *Evaluating Thoughts and Beliefs* and principle 10: *Social Support's Import*. Some of the items on the Cognitive-Behavioral Coping Skills subscale specifically address cognitive restructuring (item 16), cognitive dissonance (Festinger, 1957) regarding anti-Black racism (item 15), and cognitive-oriented appraisals or perceptions of social support as it pertains to dealing with anti-Black racism (items

12, 14, and 17). Rodgerick "Strongly Agree[ed]" with item 16, suggesting that he may already have some insight regarding the utility of reframing his thoughts. Rodgerick's composite score on the CuTS, Cognitive-Behavioral Coping Skills subscale, would be further discussed during his biopsychosocial assessment to tease out some specific interventions that may have utility for Rodgerick's GAD and concurrent psychosocial problems associated with anti-Black racial injustice.

5.7.15.3 Willingness to Seek Treatment for Cultural Trauma—CuTS Subscale (Gregory & Tucker Edmonds, 2024a)

The Willingness to Seek Treatment for Cultural Trauma subscale is a two-item subscale (composite score range between 2 and 14) that provides a basic quantitative estimate of the Black client's willingness to discuss cultural trauma with professionals. Higher scores on this subscale are indicative of greater degrees of willingness to discuss culturally traumatic experiences or issues. Rodgerick's composite score was a 9/14, indicating some willingness to discuss issues regarding Black cultural trauma. This subscale, similar to all of the CuTS subscales, should be used in the context of the biopsychosocial assessment, collateral information from family and other service providers (provided that all ethical and legal requirements have been satisfied), and other clinically relevant information.

5.7.15.4 Tripartite Police Fear—CuTS Subscale (Gregory & Tucker Edmonds, 2024a)

The Tripartite Police Fear subscale quantifies a Black individual's police fear for the Black individual themselves (in this case Rodgerick), the Black individual's fear of police as it pertains to their family members, and the individual's family members' fear of police for the client (in this case, Rodgerick's perception of his family's fear of police as it pertains to him). The Tripartite Police Fear subscale is considered a representation of structural racism and ranges between 4 and 28. Higher scores on this subscale are indicative of greater fear of police as it pertains to the individual and their family. On this subscale, Rodgerick scored a 25/28, indicating a very substantive degree of police fear for himself and his family. Regarding principle 2, *Empathy for Black Traumatic Events and Stressors*, perhaps one of the functions of the subscale could be to counter some of the potential Pollyannish beliefs that some therapists (Drakulich et al., 2023) may have as it pertains to their view of policing and Black American communities.

5.7.15.5 Resilience—CuTS Subscale (Gregory & Tucker Edmonds, 2024a)

The measurement of a Black American client's resilience supports the first principle of *Resilience and Strength of Black Americans*. The Resilience subscale of the CuTS has four items and a composite score that ranges between 4 and 28, with higher scores on the subscale being indicative of more resilience. Rodgerick's composite score was a 21/28, representing the presence of resilience as it pertains to Black racial injustice. After further discussing Rodgerick's responses in the biopsychosocial assessment, the Resilience subscale can also be used to inform Rodgerick's cognitive-behavioral case formulation. Additional factors pertaining to Rodgerick's resilience and strengths are discussed below, in the Strengths subsection of Rodgerick's biopsychosocial assessment.

5.7.16 Suicide/Homicide

Rodgerick reports that he has never attempted suicide. Rodgerick denies having any thoughts, plans, or intentions of killing himself. Rodgerick denies having any access to firearms. Rodgerick reports not having any thoughts, plans, or intentions of killing anyone.

5.7.17 Substance Use

Rodgerick denies any current substance use. Rodgerick reports that he has "never smoked anything" including cigarettes. Rodgerick denies using drugs outright. Rodgerick reports that he has had alcohol no more than three times in the last 6 months. Rodgerick states that he will typically not have more than "a few sips of beer" and reports that his alcohol use is always related to social events with acquaintances.

5.7.18 Strengths

Rodgerick brought a number of strengths to the CBT process. The strengths identified in his biopsychosocial assessment and the CuTS included the following:

1. *Family*: Loving mother, supportive siblings.
2. *Spirituality*: Belief in and knowledge of Biblical scriptures, faith.

3. *Good Candidate for CBT*: As identified by his response to the CuTS item 16 and further confirming discussion, Rodgerick demonstrated an ability to be introspective.
4. *Prosocial Educational Goals and Daily Routine*: As indicated by Rodgerick's consistent attendance in college, GPA, and part-time job.
5. *Resilience*: As initially evidenced by Rodgerick's composite score on the CuTS Resilience subscale and further support stemming from Rodgerick's biopsychosocial assessment. Take, for example, Rodgerick's statement pertaining to his ability to "thrive" despite difficult social situations.
6. *Black Identity*: Rodgerick initially appears to have a fairly stable and positive perception of his Black identity and culture. Further evidence for this is Rodgerick's report that he would like to have more Black friends and interactions with other Black people.

5.8 Review of Clinical Research Pertaining to Anxiety and Black Individuals

In accordance with principle 7, *Critical Evaluation of Clinical and other Relevant Research*, clinical research was reviewed as it pertains to CBT and Black individuals with GAD. Although the extant literature is scant, pre-experimental research specific to GAD and CBT (Markell et al., 2014) and meta-analytic CBT research including a number of anxiety diagnoses (Gregory Jr., 2019) supported the use of CBT for GAD with Rodgerick. Consistent with principle 8 (*Truth and Transparency*) and evidence-based practice (Drisko & Grady, 2015), the use of CBT with Rodgerick was discussed, including the comparative lack of external validity as it pertains to Black Americans. Rodgerick agreed to participate, realizing the CBT for GAD research was limited regarding Black external validity.

5.9 Cognitive-Behavioral Case Formulation: Black Male Exemplar with Rodgerick

Clinical information has now been obtained from Rodgerick using both a biopsychosocial assessment as well as clinically and culturally relevant scales. This information was used to draft an initial, cognitive-behavioral case formulation for Rodgerick. According to Tompkins (1997) case formulation is a theory about the psychological processes which contribute to a client's presenting issues. As stated by Persons (1989; Persons & Mooney, 1995), key aspects of the cognitive-behavioral case formulation include those manifest factors, identified as client problems and the latent psychological factors which produce the client's problems. The cognitive-behavioral case formulation used for Rodgerick is different from traditional case formulations because this case formulation includes those broader case-specific, structural factors that may potentially impact therapeutic rapport, perceptions of reality, cognitive-behavioral interventions, and clinically relevant Black social realities. Despite these social realities (macro factors which create and sustain anti-Black racial injustice) not necessarily being amenable to psychotherapeutic intervention, they have a substantial influence on the therapeutic process and therefore should be considered when working with Rodgerick and other Black clients.

5.9.1 Co-Constructing the Cognitive-Behavioral Case Conceptualization with the Black American Client

In accordance with the spirit of the RESPPECTUS principles, the cognitive-behavioral case formulation should be co-created and shared with the Black American client. Beck (2021) has previously discussed the importance of clinicians understanding their clients' realities, seeking feedback from clients, and sharing case conceptualizations with their clients. The cognitive-behavioral clinician uses their knowledge of CBT and knowledge of the client to define and integrate the various components of the case formulation. The Black American client uses their idiosyncratic and collective Black experience to co-create and modify the cognitive-behavioral case conceptualization. As with any client assessment, the case conceptualization is ongoing and will change over time. The shared co-development of the cognitive-behavioral case conceptualization should remain collaborative throughout treatment. Key aspects of Rodgerick's case conceptualization included the following components:

1. *Initial Anxiety Provoking Thoughts about Future*: Negative thinking and anticipation of bad outcomes, despite their low likelihood; catastrophic thoughts.
2. *Thoughts about Self*: Doubts his ability to effectively manage anxiety symptoms (low self-efficacy regarding coping); negative views of himself; believes that he is protected or inoculated by his worrying.
3. *Primary Emotional Concern(s):* Anxiety.
4. *Behaviors*: Avoidance of social situations, despite to desire to socially engage.
5. *Strengths/Resilience*: Introspective, history of succeeding in difficult situations, determined, strong relationship with mother, values his relationship with God, values his relationship with siblings, prosocial goals and daily activities, Black racial identity is positive, willingness to discuss cultural trauma as it relates to anxiety, currently possesses some coping skills for dealing with cultural trauma.

6. *Structural Factors that Influence Therapeutic Rapport and Client's Perceptions of Reality*: Rodgerick has concerns regarding anti-Black Racism and some pessimistic beliefs regarding structures/systems. Rodgerick has a high degree of fear regarding police as it pertains to himself and his family and a history of negative interactions with police.
7. *Cognitive-Behavioral Interventions*: Psychoeducation regarding the overall cognitive model and the cognitive model of anxiety, cognitive restructuring to identify, test, and modify thinking errors that contribute to anxiety, problem-solving to address situations that require behavioral, rather than or in addition to cognitive change, use and expand Black social network/support system.
8. *Primary Outcome Measures*: GAD-7, PHQ-9.
9. *Supplemental Outcome Information*: Client self-reported feedback.

Rodgerick was presented with a rationale for the case conceptualization. Rodgerick was informed that the cognitive-behavioral case conceptualization was an evolving document that integrated information he reported (biopsychosocial assessment and feedback from scales) into a plan to guide his cognitive-behavioral treatment. After the biopsychosocial assessment and completion of scales, the clinician collaboratively completed the cognitive-behavioral case conceptualization with Rodgerick, explaining the reasoning behind the document and asking for Roderick's input and feedback.

5.10 Cognitive-Behavioral Case Conceptualization with Black Americans: Summary

The present chapter identified and described scales which could be used in the cognitive-behavioral case conceptualization and to assess and measure progress in CBT with Black American clients. The case of Rodgerick, a young adult Black American man, was used to demonstrate an initial biopsychosocial assessment and case conceptualization using selected scales. The CuTS (Gregory & Tucker Edmonds, 2024a, 2024b) was also used to further demonstrate the scale's potential use in a clinical context. The clinical utility of the RESPPECTUS principles was also discussed in the context of cognitive-behavioral case conceptualization and treatment. Chapter 6 discusses the use of cognitive and behavioral interventions with Black clients using the RESPPECTUS principles. Chapter 6 also provides a specific application of cognitive-behavioral interventions for the case of Rodgerick.

References

Alexander, M. (2010). *The new Jim crow: Mass incarceration in the ages of colorblindness*. The New Press.

American Psychiatric Association. (2022). *Diagnostic and statistical manual of mental disorders* (5th ed., text rev.). doi:https://doi.org/10.1176/appi.books.9780890425787.

Bailey, Z. D., Krieger, N., Agénor, M., Graves, J., Linos, N., & Bassett, M. T. (2017). Structural racism and health inequities in the USA: Evidence and interventions. *Lancet, 389*(10077), 1453–1463. https://doi.org/10.1016/S0140-6736(17)30569-X

Beck, J. S. (2021). *Cognitive behavior therapy: Basics and beyond* (3rd ed.). Guilford Press.

Beck, A. T., Rush, A. J., Shaw, B. F., & Emery, G. (1979). *Cognitive therapy of depression.* Guilford Press.

Bertalanffy, L. (1969). *General systems theory: Foundation, development, application.* George Braziller.

Bowleg, L., English, D., del Rio-Gonzalez, A. M., Burkholder, G. J., Teti, M., & Tschann, J. M. (2016). Measuring the pros and cons of what it means to be a Black man: Development and validation of the Black Men's Experiences Scale (BMES). *Psychology of Men and Masculinity, 17*(2), 177–188. https://doi.org/10.1037/men0000026

Briggs, H. E., Huggins-Hoyt, K. Y., Teasley, M. L., & Hopps, J. G. (2022). Poverty or racism?: Determinants of disproportionality and disparity for African American/Black Children in Child Welfare. *Research on Social Work Practice, 32*(5), 533–538. https://doi.org/10.1177/10497315221076830

Bryne, B. M. (2016). *Structural equation modeling with Amos: Basic concepts, applications, and programming* (3rd ed.). Taylor & Francis.

Carter, R. T., & Muchow, C. (2017). Construct validity of the Race-Based Traumatic Stress Symptom Scale and tests of measurement equivalence. *Psychological Trauma: Theory, Research, Practice, and Policy, 9*(6), 688–695. https://doi.org/10.1037/tra0000256

Carter, R. T., Mazzula, S., Victoria, R., Vazquez, R., Hall, S., Smith, S., Sant-Barket, S., Forsyth, J., Bazelais, K., & Williams, B. (2013). Initial development of the Race-Based Traumatic Stress Symptom Scale: Assessing the emotional impact of racism. *Psychological Trauma: Theory, Research, Practice, and Policy, 5*(1), 1–9. https://doi.org/10.1037/a0025911

Carter, R. T., Muchow, C., & Pieterse, A. L. (2018). Construct, predictive validity, and measurement equivalence of the Race-Based Traumatic Stress Symptom Scale for Black Americans. *Traumatology, 24*(1), 8–16. https://doi.org/10.1037/trm0000128

Cavalhieri, K. E., Greer, T. M., Hawkins, D., Choi, H., Hardy, C., & Heavner, E. (2023). The effects of online and institutional racism on the mental health of African Americans. *Cultural Diversity and Ethnic Minority Psychology*. https://doi.org/10.1037/cdp0000585

Corley, N. A., & Young, S. M. (2018). Is social work still racist? A content analysis of recent literature. *Social Work, 63*(4), 317–326. https://doi.org/10.1093/sw/swy042

Cronbach, L. J. (1951). Coefficient alpha and the internal structure of tests. *Psychometrika, 16*(3), 297–334. https://doi.org/10.1007/BF02310555

Diener, E., Emmons, R. A., Larsen, R. J., & Griffin, S. (1985). The satisfaction with life scale. *Journal of Personality Assessment, 49*(1), 71. https://doi.org/10.1207/s15327752jpa4901_13

Drakulich, K., Rodriguez-Whitney, E., & Robles, J. (2023). Why white Americans more frequently fail to view the Police critically. *Abstract Du Bois Review: Social Science Research on Race, 20*(1), 57–88. https://doi.org/10.1017/S1742058X22000133

Drisko, J., & Grady, M. (2015). Evidence-based practice in social work: A contemporary perspective. *Clinical Social Work Journal, 43*(3), 274–282. https://doi.org/10.1007/s10615-015-0548-z

Edwards, F., Lee, H., & Esposito, M. (2019). Risk of being killed by police use of force in the United States by age, race-ethnicity, and sex. *Proceedings of the National Academy of Sciences of the United States of America, 116*(34), 16793–16798. https://doi.org/10.1073/pnas.1821204116

Engel, G. L. (1977). The need for a new medical model: A challenge for biomedicine. *Science, 196*(4286), 129–136. https://doi.org/10.1126/science.847460

Festinger, L. (1957). *A theory of cognitive dissonance*. Stanford University Press.

Forsyth, J. M., & Carter, R. T. (2014). Development and preliminary validation of the Racism-Related Coping Scale. *Psychological Trauma: Theory, Research, Practice, and Policy, 6*(6), 632–643. https://doi.org/10.1037/a0036702

Gregory, V. L., Jr. (2019). Cognitive-behavioral therapy for anxious symptoms in persons of African descent: A meta-analysis. *Journal of Social Service Research, 45*(1), 87–101. https://doi.org/10.1080/01488376.2018.1479344

Gregory, V. L., Jr., & Tucker Edmonds, J. L. (2023). The racial pandemic experienced by Black American men: Cognitive-behavioral and structural implications. *American Journal of Orthopsychiatry, 93*(1), 1–16. https://doi.org/10.1037/ort0000651

Gregory, V. L., Jr., & Tucker Edmonds, J. L. (2024a). Cultural Trauma Scale: Psychometric evaluation of Black men's beliefs, emotions, and coping. *Psychological Trauma: Theory, Research, Practice, and Policy, 16*(8), 1329–1337. https://doi.org/10.1037/tra0001607

Gregory, V. L., Jr., & Tucker Edmonds, J. L. (2024b). Cultural Trauma Scale (CuTS): Parsimonious principal component analysis, independent Black American male sample. *Journal of Aggression, Maltreatment and Trauma, 33*(3), 369–386. https://doi.org/10.1080/10926771.2023.2256741

Gurpinar-Morgan, A., Murray, C., & Beck, A. (2014). Ethnicity and the therapeutic relationship: Views of young people accessing cognitive behavioural therapy. *Mental Health, Religion and Culture, 17*(7), 714–725. https://doi.org/10.1080/13674676.2014.903388

Kirkinis, K., Pieterse, A. L., Martin, C., Agiliga, A., & Brownell, A. (2021). Racism, racial discrimination, and trauma: a systematic review of the social science literature. *Ethnicity & Health, 26*(3), 392–412. https://doi.org/10.1080/13557858.2018.1514453

Kroenke, K., Spitzer, R. L., & Williams, J. B. W. (2001). The PHQ-9. *Journal of General Internal Medicine, 16*(9), 606–613. https://doi.org/10.1046/j.1525-1497.2001.016009606.x

Lyons, J. S., & Walton, B. A. (2007). *Adult Needs and Strength Assessment (ANSA): Indiana ANSA manual, version 2*. The Praed Foundation.

Markell, H. M., Newman, M. G., Gallop, R., Gibbons, M. B., Rickels, K., & Crits-Christoph, P. (2014). Combined medication and CBT for generalized anxiety disorder with African American participants: Reliability and validity of assessments and preliminary outcomes. *Behavior Therapy, 45*(4), 495–506. https://doi.org/10.1016/j.beth.2014.02.008

Mouzon, D. M., & McLean, J. S. (2017). Internalized racism and mental health among African-Americans, US-born Caribbean Blacks, and foreign-born Caribbean Blacks. *Ethnicity and Health, 22*(1), 36–48. https://doi.org/10.1080/13557858.2016.1196652

Nadal, K. L. (2011). The racial and ethnic microaggressions scale (REMS): Construction, reliability, and validity. *Journal of Counseling Psychology, 58*(4), 470–480. https://doi.org/10.1037/a0025193

Nichols, M. P., & Davis, S. D. (2017). *Family therapy: Concepts and methods* (11th ed.). Pearson.

Nunnally, J. C., & Bernstein, I. H. (1994). *Psychometric theory* (3rd ed.). McGraw-Hill.

Persons, J. B. (1989). *Cognitive therapy in practice: A case formulation approach*. Norton.

Persons, J. B. (2008). *The case formulation approach to cognitive-behavior therapy*. The Guilford Press.

Persons, J. B., & Mooney, K. A. (1995). Interrater reliability of cognitive-behavioral case formulations. *Cognitive Therapy and Research, 19*(1), 21–34. https://doi.org/10.1007/BF02229674

Persons, J. B., Davidson, J., & Tompkins, M. A. (2001). *Essential components of cognitive-behavior therapy for depression*. American Psychological Association.

Pieterse, A. L., Roberson, K. L., Garcia, R., & Carter, R. T. (2023). Racial discrimination and trauma symptoms: Further support for the Race-Based Traumatic Stress Symptom Scale. *Cultural Diversity and Ethnic Minority Psychology, 29*(3), 332–338. https://doi.org/10.1037/cdp0000544

Rosenberg, M. (1989). *Society and the adolescent self-image*. Wesleyan University Press.

Shedler, J. (2010). The efficacy of psychodynamic psychotherapy. *American Psychologist, 65*(2), 98–109. https://doi.org/10.1037/a0018378

Spitzer, R. L., Kroenke, K., Williams, J. B., & Swinson, R. P. (2006). The GAD-7 scale was accurate for diagnosing generalized anxiety disorder. *Evidence Based Medicine, 11*(6), 184.

Tompkins, M. A. (1997). Case formulation in cognitive-behavioral therapy. In R. Leahy (Ed.), *Practicing cognitive therapy: A guide to interventions* (pp. 37–59). Jason Aronson.

Utsey, S. O. (1999). Development and validation of a short form of the Index of Race-Related Stress (IRRS)-brief version. *Measurement and Evaluation in Counseling and Development, 32*(3), 149. https://doi.org/10.1080/07481756.1999.12068981

Utsey, S. O., & Ponterotto, J. G. (1996). Development and validation of the index of race-related stress (IRRS). *Journal of Counseling Psychology, 43*(4), 490. https://doi.org/10.1037/0022-0167.43.4.490

Wallace, C. J., Lecomte, T., Wilde, J., & Liberman, R. P. (2001). CASIG: A consumer-centered assessment for planning individualized treatment and evaluating program outcomes. *Schizophrenia Research, 50*, 105–119. https://doi.org/10.1016/S0920-9964(00)00068-2

Walton, B. A., & Kim, H.-W. (2018). Validating a behavioral health instrument for adults: Exploratory factor analysis. *Journal of Social Service Research, 44*(2), 249–265. https://doi.org/10.1080/01488376.2018.1442897

Williams, M. T., Printz, D. M. B., & DeLapp, R. C. T. (2018). Assessing racial trauma with the Trauma Symptoms of Discrimination Scale. *Psychology of Violence, 8*(6), 735–747. https://doi.org/10.1037/vio0000212

Williams, M. T., Osman, M., Gallo, J., Pereira, D. P., Gran-Ruaz, S., Strauss, D., Lester, L., George, J. R., Edelman, J., & Litman, L. (2022). A clinical scale for the assessment of racial trauma. *Practice Innovations, 7*(3), 223–240. https://doi.org/10.1037/pri0000178

Williams-Washington, K. N., & Mills, C. P. (2018). African American historical trauma: Creating an inclusive measure. *Journal of Multicultural Counseling and Development, 46*(4), 246–263. https://doi.org/10.1002/jmcd.12113

Chapter 6
Cognitive-Behavioral Interventions: Integrating RESPPECTUS Principles

6.1 Cognitive Restructuring with Black Americans

6.1.1 Objective Black Reality and the Social Construction of Black Reality

Cognitive-behavioral therapy (CBT) typically maintains that there is an objective reality, and work in CBT consists of examining the evidence and processing the meaning of this new information (Dobson, 2012). This CBT-embraced objective reality is indeed compatible with structurally informed CBT for Black Americans. Throughout American history, Black Americans have collectively, correctly appraised their value as human beings and objectively compared their value to their social status, social progress, rights, and available opportunities in American society. Throughout American history, when there was a perceived discrepancy between Black Americans' collective self-appraisals and available rights and liberties, this discrepancy has been a catalyst for behavioral and social change. The individual and collective self-appraisals by Black Americans speak to Black Americans' ability to be introspective and to make positive changes that suggest a cultural and historical compatibility with the CBT-embraced notion of an objective reality.

Regarding Black Americans and CBT, the social construction of reality should also be considered (Berger & Luckmann, 1966). The social construction of reality includes the process by which knowledge, which may vary by group, culture, and subgroups within cultures, becomes recognized as real and independently valid. However, Berger and Luckmann maintain that knowledge may best be understood or determined by the collective agreement, of what is real or true, despite the objective reality. Given this definition of knowledge and its relationship to objective truth, it becomes easier to understand how what may be considered true or valid in one culture may lack truth or credibility in another culture. This difference in what is true stems from a collective consensus around viewing the same events or situations

V. L. Gregory, Jr., *Cognitive-Behavioral Therapy with Black Americans*,
https://doi.org/10.1007/978-3-032-01666-9_6

differently in another culture, hence the social construction of reality. The stance of this book is consistent with that of Alford and Beck (1997), which states that CBT adopts both an objective reality and a socially constructed reality. These dual realities have implications for both the Black clients receiving CBT and the clinicians providing CBT.

6.1.2 The Cognitive-Behavioral Clinician's View of Black American Culture

Culture has been defined as beliefs held by a specific group of people that influence their behavior (Edberg, 2022). This definition of culture is particularly useful because this cognitive perspective shares similarities with the basic cognitive model (Beck, 2021) that is used to guide CBT. Black Americans have unique African, ancestral identities as well as historical and contemporary experiences in America that simultaneously and interactively shape the strengths, challenges, and distinctive attributes of Black culture. Black American culture has been a strong force in shifting the larger American culture. There are examples, including how Black Americans' fights for civil rights have changed policy and public opinion regarding how Black culture is viewed in America and across the world. Many groups experiencing various forms of injustice have used the self-affirming beliefs and social change methods used in Black culture to affirm their own respective cultural identities. Black American culture has also influenced various aspects of popular American culture by providing an archetype for what is fashionable and in vogue (Gregory & Tucker Edmonds, 2023). As is true for other cultures in America, different aspects of Black culture have a range of influences on clinical outcomes that CBT will be used to address. For example, a qualitative study with Black adults, asked participants how Black culture may promote or inhibit substance use recovery for Black individuals (Gregory et al., 2025). Participants noted strengths of the Black culture that promoted substance use recovery, including a shared sense of black struggle and achievement, positive racial identity, and spirituality among other factors. Participants in this study noted that factors which stifle Black recovery from substance use include being deluged with images of substance use and violence in Black popular media. Recognizing the positive and powerful influence of Black culture on Black individuals and the broader American culture is consistent with the first principle of CBT with Black Americans, *Resilience and Strength of Black Americans*. This principle underscores the importance of not viewing Black American culture in a negative and deficit-based manner.

Despite the helping professions being typically viewed as bringing individuals who have a strong commitment to social justice, a study has shown anti-Black racism and anti-working class discrimination in clients' ability to access therapy appointments (Kugelmass, 2016). Beyond availability, once Black clients receive services, clinicians having negative views of Black culture will ultimately undermine therapeutic rapport with Black clients. Clinicians viewing Black culture from a nuanced and strength-based perspective (principle 1, *Resilience and Strength of Black Americans*), is a prerequisite for the effectiveness of CBT with Black Americans. As alluded to in principle 9, *Uniqueness of Each Black Individual*, Black individuals are multidimensional; therefore, narrow or stereotypical views of Black culture is fundamentally flawed and will certainly compromise cognitive-behavioral therapy with Black Americans. Negative and stereotypical views of Black Americans will inevitably corrupt the cognitive-behavioral clinician's case conceptualization, diagnosis, perceived credibility of information coming from Black clients, verbal and written communication to and about Black clients, and efforts to identify and challenge thoughts and beliefs that Black clients report in CBT.

6.1.3 Cognitive-Behavioral Therapist's Beliefs About Black Clients

Black clients receiving treatment may have a socially constructed reality that is different from the socially constructed reality of their cognitive-behavioral therapist. The perspective-shifting process, inherent in CBT, is relevant for CBT with Black Americans in a number of ways. First, it is possible that a clinician who may have a false and negative view of Black people may change in response to substantive evidence to the contrary. Berger and Luckmann (1966) also discussed how perceptions of reality change when confronted with experiential evidence to the contrary. The question then becomes what harm may be done to the Black client and/or community as the clinician's Black myths or stereotypical perceptions are slowly eroded away through experiential evidence to the contrary. As stated before, a clinician's negative beliefs about Black people and Black culture could result in: inaccurate case conceptualizations, misdiagnoses, viewing the Black client as being an incredible source of information, negative verbal and written communication to and about Black clients, biased mandated reporting to third parties, and/or ineffective or detrimental cognitive restructuring resulting in the clinician's imposition of values or ontological perspective on the Black client. These costs and their implications are too high; therefore, addressing CBT clinicians' thoughts about Black people and Black culture must be addressed proactively, at the educational, supervision, and societal levels. Although actions should be taken to address cognitive-behavioral clinicians who have negative beliefs about Black people and culture, doing so purely in a reactive stance permits harm to be done to Black individuals, families, and communities.

6.1.4 Black Client's Beliefs About Cognitive-Behavioral Therapists

Rapport-relevant thoughts or beliefs, by the Black client, about the cognitive-behavioral therapist could enhance or undermine rapport building and trust that is necessary for CBT to be effective. It is possible that, given long-standing anti-Black structural racism, disproportionate anti-Black violence, and other structural and institutional factors that diminish the structural trust held by Black communities, the therapeutic relationship with both non-Black and Black CBT clinicians could be jeopardized. Several studies have empirically documented how perceptions of structural racism (Gregory et al., in press) and subsidiary social aspects of structural racism (Scott & Davis, 2006) are empirically associated with negative beliefs about mental health treatment for Black individuals. For a non-Black cognitive-behavioral therapist, there may be trust issues that hinder the Black client's introspection, vulnerability, and willingness to share with a non-Black therapist. As it pertains to Black trauma and its structural determinants, Black clients may not believe that a White clinician will understand or empathize with their interpretation of race-related events or overall worldview (Gregory et al., 2025). Research has supported the notion that Black therapists, regardless of therapeutic allegiance, use their identity, experience, and understanding of Black communities to help them relate to their Black clientele (Goode-Cross & Grim, 2016). A race-related lack of trust for White or non-Black cognitive-behavioral clinicians could hinder the full disclosure of thoughts and beliefs that underlie various emotions and behaviors, thereby decreasing the functionality of cognitive-behavioral interventions. If the CBT clinician is Black, a Black client with acknowledged or unacknowledged, internalized anti-Black racism may present some factors which could be contrary to therapeutic rapport with a Black cognitive-behavioral clinician. For Black clients who have internalized anti-Black racism, their reasons for coming to treatment may or may not be related to internalized anti-Black racism, thereby making the development and maintenance of therapeutic rapport more challenging.

6.1.5 Therapeutic Rapport and Cognitive Restructuring with Black American Clients

Within the context of therapeutic rapport, Beck and associates (1979) state that the clinician and client work together to decide to what extent the client's perceptions and interpretations meet basic standards of objectivity. Judith Beck (2021) later referred to this process as Collaborative Empiricism. Collaborative empiricism is the process by which the clinician works with the Black client to evaluate the correctness of his thoughts (Beck, 2021). As it pertains to the identification, systematic evaluation, and replacement of maladaptive thoughts and beliefs held by Black clients and their unique experiences in America, a racial tension can exist regarding what is a cognitive distortion that requires cognitive restructuring. For example, in the case of Rodgerick, his social situations in high school and college were associated with anxiety-provoking thoughts, such as he would be alone in the future. While this thought and interpretation of events could very well be an Overgeneralizing cognitive distortion (Burns, 1989), there is an inherent challenge to harmonizing Rodgerick's Black social reality with the productive and useful change that may occur via cognitive restructuring. Using cognitive restructuring, regarding race-related events and their consequent psychological trauma, while maintaining a good therapeutic rapport, could be difficult. The difficulty may in-part arise from the Black client's potential perception that a White therapist has no insight or credibility to even begin guiding him in challenging the validity of his thoughts. Rodgerick may hold the belief that, as a Black man (client), he lives in a world that is fundamentally different from his White clinician's world.

Beck (1976) very wisely discussed the potential for the clinician to inadvertently impose his values on the client. Beck maintained that a thought could be considered a cognitive distortion if the clinician and client have a consensus that the client's cognition hinders functioning and/or contentment. The realities and perceptions of events of Black American clients and non-Black or Black clinicians can be vastly different. This difference can potentially, although not necessarily, be an obstacle to therapeutic rapport and the effective implementation of CBT with Black American clients. These tensions and difficulties regarding cognitive restructuring and therapeutic rapport underscore the importance of principles 2 (*Empathy for Black Traumatic Events and Stressors* and principles), 6 (*Evaluating Thoughts and Beliefs*), and 8 (*Truth and Transparency*). Later in this chapter the RESPPECTUS principles are used to illustrate how cognitive restructuring was used with Rodgerick to address his thoughts as they pertained to anxiety associated with his culturally specific situation.

6.1.6 The Cognitive Model

Central to cognitive-behavioral interventions is the cognitive model. The cognitive model maintains that misperceptions or misinterpretations of events lead to emotional disorders (Beck, 1976). The cognitive model provides clients with the basic framework upon which cognitive interventions are used. The cognitive model serves as an explanation for how thoughts influence mood and behavior (Beck, 1976) and a rationale for interventions in cognitive-behavioral therapy (Beck et al., 1979). Educating Black American clients in the cognitive model can be done using didactic methods. As described in Chap. 2, with the case example of Serita, didactic approaches to educating Black clients in the cognitive model may beneficially incorporate several approaches. One approach to teaching the cognitive model is Ellis's ABCD model (1994, pgs. 78–79): Activating Event (A), Beliefs about the Event (B), Consequences (emotional and behavioral) due to the Beliefs (C), and

Disputation of the Beliefs (D). Ellis's model highlights the importance of Beliefs mediating events and emotional consequences. Ellis emphasized the relationship between irrational beliefs and negative emotional and behavioral outcomes and pointed to the necessity of changing Beliefs to alter emotional and behavioral consequences (C). Ellis has Socratic questions that are used to aid in the Disputation of maladaptive beliefs. Another traditional approach to teaching the cognitive model is the Thought Record (Beck et al., 1979). The Though Record, similar to Ellis's ABCD model, emphasizes the role of thoughts/beliefs in determining emotions and behavioral outcomes; however, the thought record can also include metrics to assess the subjective, quantitative, pre–post impact of challenging the identified thought (Beck, 2021). Both the ABCD model and Thought Record illustrate the connections between events, beliefs, emotions/behaviors, and both involve the use of empirical, functional, philosophical, and other types of Socratic questions to evaluate potentially negative beliefs (Bishop, 2001). Another method for teaching the cognitive model and retrospectively demonstrating the link between events, thoughts/beliefs, and emotions is the functional analysis (Carroll, 1998). A functional analysis is often used to analyze substance-related triggers, thoughts and emotions, responses (substance use), and positive and negative consequences. The positive and negative consequences of substance use, obtained from the functional analysis, can be used to illustrate the biphasic nature of substance use (Marlatt, 1985) and inform cognitive interventions to challenge substance-related thoughts.

6.1.7 Didactic Explanation of the Cognitive Model: A Structurally Informed Perspective with Black American Clients

There are several ways in which the cognitive model can be effectively explained in a culturally responsive manner for Black American clients. The cognitive model, regardless of the method that is employed to explain its components (ABCD model, Thought Record, etc.), should use examples that the Black client can relate to. Solely relying on clinician-perceived social norms of Black American culture is flawed and contrary to principle 9, *Uniqueness of Each Black Individual*. Principle 9 maintains that Black individuals are heterogeneous in their beliefs, values, experiences, and countless other factors. Therefore, illustrating the ABCD model by relying on examples of situations that are stereotypically "Black" can be counterproductive to the didactic explanation of the cognitive model (teaching) and the development and maintenance of therapeutic rapport with the Black client.

In the author's work with Black Americans using CBT, the following steps were used to explain the cognitive model as a rationale for cognitive-behavioral interventions and teach the client about how their thoughts impact their emotions and behaviors:

1. **A Rationale for CBT Using a Didactic Method**: A rationale for CBT was provided by explaining each component of the ABCD model (Ellis, 1994) and the ABCD model's implications for the interventions that would be used in work with the Black client.
2. **A Culturally Relevant Example**: As the therapist, the author would give a culturally relevant example of the ABCD model, using a situation (A), thought (B), and emotions (C) based on information provided from the client's most recent situation/issue, initial assessment and/or cognitive-behavioral case conceptualization.
3. **Questions for Clarification about the Cognitive Model**: The Black client would be asked if they had any questions about the ABCD model. If the client asked questions, the questions would be answered.
4. **Client Summarization of the Cognitive Model**: The Black client would then be asked to summarize the ABCD model and its implications for the interventions we would be using.
5. **Feedback on the Client's Summarization of the Cognitive Model**: The client's summary allowed the author, as the therapist, the opportunity to both clarify and affirm the client for their correct understanding of the ABCD model and its implications for cognitive-behavioral intervention.
6. **The Contributing Role of Structural Issues and Policy**: In accordance with principles 3 (*Structural Racism—Influences on Presenting Problems, Rapport, and Therapy*) and 5 (*Policy Change*) policy may be discussed. Structural racism and/or police may be discussed, depending on the nature of the client's reasons for coming to treatment of the specific event (A) or thought (B) being discussed.
7. **Continued Reinforcement of the Cognitive Model and Structural Intervention throughout CBT**: The cognitive model is continually discussed and reinforced throughout the author's work with the Black client via teaching new cognitive and behavioral interventions, setting homework assignments, reviewing homework assignments, and adding a cognitive framework to various problematic situations the Black client experiences. As necessary for each Black client, the clinically relevant structural aspects of the client's presenting problems are acknowledged (principle 3, *Structural Racism—Influences on Presenting Problems, Rapport, and Therapy*) and translated into treatment relevant interventions. Clinically relevant structural interventions could include case or class advocacy on behalf of the client, teaching the client to advocate for themselves (assertiveness and communication skills), linking the client to supportive agencies that address structural level interventions [case management] and/or other relevant resources.

Similar to traditional CBT, client thoughts that create negative moods and behaviors are categorized. These categorizations of thoughts are often diagnosis-dependent, but not always. In the case of Rodgerick and his diagnosis of Generalized Anxiety Disorder, cognitive distortions identified by Burns (1989) were discussed as various ways to categorize the thoughts (B) that may contribute to Rodgerick's anxiety (C). These cognitive distortions included: Overgeneralization, Mental Filter, Discounting the Positives, and Emotional Reasoning. Perhaps the biggest difference between the traditional didactic explanation of the cognitive model, compared to the structurally informed CBT approach, is that the latter takes into account the roles of structural racism (principle 3: *Structural Racism—Influences on Presenting Problems, Rapport, and Therapy*) and policy (principle 5: *Policy Change*) in contributing to and addressing the client's issue, respectively. Another difference with structurally informed CBT is the identification and evaluation of cognitive distortions (B) related to structural injustice events (A). Below, four types of cognitive distortions related to Black social injustice are identified and defined. Via identifying and acknowledging the impact of larger social forces on the Black client's problems and their treatment implications, the client is validated by not making internal attributions for factors which are structural in nature. The use of cognitive-behavioral interventions during therapy is also streamlined to address only those factors which are truly best addressed at the micro (rather than macro) level.

6.1.8 Anti-Black Structural Injustice: Cognitive Distortions and Consequences

Cognitive distortions are errors in thinking, which are contrary to reality, and result in emotional disorders (Beck, 1976) and counterproductive behavior (Beck, 2021). Black Americans have structural forces that impact their individual being, families, communities, opportunities for advancement, and social environment. The impact of these structural forces (activating events) also includes cognitive distortions that arise based on the Black individual's distorted interpretations of these events. Typical cognitive distortions of structural injustice events include:

1. **Diminished Self-Efficacy (B_1)**: The devaluation of the Black individual's self-perceived ability to overcome anti-Black social injustice can compound other negative, disorder-specific belief systems. For example, research examining Black individuals' reasons for substance use (Gregory et al., 2025) found relief-oriented beliefs (Beck et al., 1993) about substance use that intersected with negative experiences with and/or beliefs about structural racism.
   (a) This may involve an externalized locus of control regarding anti-Black social injustice.
2. **Internalized Anti-Black Racism (B_2)**: The adoption and internalization of negative beliefs about Black people that are present in the broader American society.
   (a) This is commonly referred to as internalized racism (Pyke, 2010).
3. **Detrimental Distrust of Systems (B_3)**: Omnibus negative beliefs about American structures that result in a distrust of systems (emotional consequence)

and refusal to engage in systems and/or civic opportunities (behavioral consequence) that may potentially correct anti-Black social injustice and Black healthcare disparities. The cyclic nature of distrust of systems that deteriorate participation in macro interventions to address social injustice and health disparities has been previously discussed (Gregory & Clary, 2022).

(a) This cognitive distortion has shown up in basic research that demonstrates a theoretical relationship between Black men's distrust of American systems (systems which could be helpful) and negative perceptions of healthcare systems (Gregory & Tucker Edmonds, 2023).
(b) There is also an empirical relationship that shows as Black men's Tripartite Police Fear increases, their negative perceptions of mental healthcare systems increase (Gregory et al., in press).

4. **The Futility of Positive Change for Self and/or Other Blacks Individuals ($\mathbf{B_4}$)**: These beliefs have in common, the assertion that progress or positive change for Black individuals and/or the Black collective in America is not possible.

   (a) Sophisticated, nonclinical, theoretical discussions, more or less related to this concept are noted in literature pertaining to Afro-pessimism (Gordon, 2023).

These types of misinterpretations of events or cognitive distortions could catalyze and/or exacerbate mental health disorders and symptoms. These cognitive distortions, related to structural racism, can also deter or complicate engagement and retention in CBT and other mental health treatment.

6.1.9 Cognitive Restructuring with Black Clients

Once the client has a substantive understanding of the cognitive model, cognitive restructuring can be used to aid the Black client in objectively evaluating thoughts within the structural context that the Black client lives in. Socratic questions can be used to evaluate or challenge cognitive distortions along empirical, functional, philosophical, and other dimensions (Bishop, 2001). The type of Socratic question that is used to evaluate a Black client's cognitive distortion would depend on the suspected type of faulty thinking which may be underlying the thought or belief. The type of Socratic question will also depend on the client's unique clinical needs and the specific situation at hand. Below, culturally relevant empirical, functional, philosophical, and action-oriented Socratic questions are discussed with regard to Black Americans.

6.1.10 *Evidence For and Against the Thought or Belief*

The empirical examination of a thought or belief can also include the objective evidence that supports and diminishes the thought or belief (Beck, 2021). Clients typically have immediate knowledge of the evidence that is believed to support a maladaptive thought or belief. Evidence against maladaptive beliefs of Black Americans may be found by considering spirituality as well as Black identity, family, and community.

6.1.10.1 Spirituality

Given the prevalence of the Christian faith in the Black community (Pew Research Center, 2021), there are a number of ways in which the evidence question can be culturally modified to draw a greater distinction between the distorted thought and the spiritual evidence which does not support it. The first principle (*Resilience and Strength of Black Americans*) calls for CBT clinicians to search for resilience and strengths within and around Black clients that can be mobilized in the use of cognitive-behavioral interventions. If the Black client already has spiritual or religious beliefs, these beliefs can be used as a resource for identifying evidence to the contrary of a maladaptive thought. A knowledge of the Black client's religious or spiritual background can be gained through the initial and ongoing assessments, as well as direct questions on the subject matter. Socratic questions could be asked that evoke the spiritual or religious content as evidence to counter a maladaptive thought or belief (B). For example, "*What spiritual or religious beliefs do you have that may be considered as evidence against this thought*?"

In response to structural racism in America, Black Americans have used religion/spiritualty and places of worship to affirm their Black identity, build their faith, and advance social justice (Pew Research Center, 2021). Based on research conducted by the Pew Center, Black Americans predominantly identify with some form of Christianity, such as protestant (66%), Catholic (6%), or other Christian religious affiliation (3%). Three percent of Black Americans have a religion that is not Christian. For Black Americans, religious strengths or resources include individual and collective prayer, scriptures, social gatherings, and faith (Gregory & Tucker Edmonds, 2023). Gregory and Tucker Edmonds have previously documented the utility of both spirituality and cognitive change for Black American men dealing with racial injustice. For Black Americans belonging to Christian faiths, there are Biblical scriptures (New International Version Holy Bible, 2011) that underscore topics which are foundational to CBT interventions. For example, some CBT compatible scriptures that can be used to identify evidence contrary to a distorted thought include:

1. The Importance of Changing Thinking:
   (a) "… whatever is true, whatever is noble, whatever is right, whatever is pure, whatever is lovely, whatever is admirable—if anything is excellent or praiseworthy—think about such things." Philippians, 4:8 (p. 1181).

2. Biblical "evidence" to the contrary of anxiety:
   (a) "Do not be anxious about anything, but in everything, by prayer and petition, with thanksgiving, present your requests to God …," Philippians, 4:6 (p. 1181).
   (b) "For the Spirit God gave us does not make us timid, but gives us power, love and self-discipline." 2 Timothy 1: 7 (p. 1197).
3. Recalling "evidence" from past positive experiences with God:
   (a) "Your servant has killed both the lion and the bear; this uncircumcised Philistine will be like one of them, because he has defied the armies of the living God." 1 Samuel 17: 36 (p. 285).
4. Reframing via meaning-making:
   (a) "… For I know the plans I have for you," declares the Lord, "plans to proser you and not harm you, plans to give you hope and a future …" Jeremiah 29:11 (p. 785–786).
   (b) "And we know that in all things God works for the good of those who love him, …" Romans 8:28, (p. 1133).

There are a vast number of scriptures that have relevance for finding evidence to the contrary of a negative thought; far too numerous to exhaustively list here. The aforementioned are simply examples of how specific scriptures may be applicable to finding religious or spiritual evidence to the contrary of a maladaptive belief or thought. To reiterate, the utilization of scriptures to find evidence to the contrary of a maladaptive belief will depend upon the Black client's predetermined religious beliefs as well as the conduct of an initial assessment that includes an exploration of the client's religious and spiritual background. It should be noted that simply because a Black client reports being a Christian, it does not necessarily mean that the client will be comfortable with using scriptures or other spiritual aspects to aid in cognitive restructuring. Cognitive-behavioral clinicians may simply ask in advance about the Black client's comfort level with discussing spiritual or religious issues during treatment and cognitive restructuring. Given Roderick's initial and ongoing assessments and his case-conceptualization, scripture-based Socratic questions to find evidence to the contrary were appropriate with Rodgerick.

6.1.10.2 Black Identity, Family, and Community

Consistent with Principle 1 (*Resilience and Strength of Black Americans*) Black cultural identity, family, and community can be outstanding resources to identify evidence to the contrary of maladaptive thoughts and beliefs. Black culture, history, family, and community may be strengths which can aid some Black clients in finding evidence that contradicts a maladaptive thought or belief. Meta-analytic research has shown a positive relationship between Black identity and Black well-being (Smith & Silva, 2011). Smith and Silva have discussed the clinical utility of the relationship between ethnic identity and well-being. As referenced earlier, the BLAC model (Turner et al., 2022) also highlights the utility of Black identity in fostering personal growth and positive change. To the extent to which Black American clients have internalized Black cultural and historical achievements as part of their collective and personal identity, these Black cultural advancements may be used as evidence to the contrary of negative perceptions. Conversely, advances made by the collective Black culture may also serve as *Evidence For* new alternative thoughts and beliefs that emerge out of cognitive restructuring efforts. As it pertains to a thought that precedes cultural hopelessness, questions such as "*Based on Black progress that has been made in this country, what evidence may be used to show positive change is possible*?" (D) may be used to identify evidence to the contrary.

Research on Black cultural trauma has documented the importance of Black family and community in coping with racial injustice (Gregory & Tucker Edmonds, 2023, 2024a, 2024b). In occupational, educational, residential, medical, and other settings where Black Americans are racially secluded (A), negative thoughts and empathic isolation may occur. Empathic isolation is an emotion that is associated with the absence of, or minimal empathy being expressed by others in society (Joe et al., 2019). Socratic questions regarding evidence against not being empathically supported would not be useful. However, negative self or future-oriented perceptions (B) drawn from such events are prime targets for cognitive intervention/Socratic questions (D). For example, Rodgerick reported believing "he will probably never have an active or rewarding dating life" (B) and this belief created anxiety (C). Rodgerick's overgeneralizing thought was one example of a cognitive distortion associated with structural injustice (impossibility of progress or change for self and/or other Black individuals). Rodgerick stated that evidence for this belief included the fact that he could not find anyone Black to go to the prom with in high school. Rodgerick was asked, "Considering your family, community, or other social networks, what evidence can you find that challenges this belief?" (D). As evidence against this belief, Rodgerick noted that:

- He has family that are married or have long-term relationships with other Black individuals despite living in racially homogenous environments,
- He has family members and friends who have used online dating to find other long-term positive relationships,
- Some people he knows have used church and social networking to meet other Black people despite living in predominantly White locations.

After reviewing the evidence for and against the belief (B: "I will probably never have an active or rewarding dating life"), Rodgerick concluded that the evidence against the belief was stronger, yet there would be some work required to obtain the relationship that he wanted. This additional work would be addressed using the problem-solving model (principle 4, *Problem-Solving*).

6.1.11 Reframing Using Psychoeducation and Alternative Explanations: Stigma Regarding Black Mental Illness

Rodgerick had reported that receiving services from "a mental health treatment center would be more appropriate for other people and not someone like me." After further follow-up questions regarding Rodgerick's thoughts about mental illness and its meaning for him within his social and cultural context, Rodgerick reported thinking that his receiving treatment from a mental health center further accentuated and supported his anxiety-related thoughts about him being "not good enough" and less competent. Rodgerick's stigmatizing thought was indicative of Labeling (Burns, 1989).

6.1.11.1 Psychoeducation

Psychoeducation was first used to destigmatize the role of Rodgerick receiving mental health services. Psychoeducation has benefits for mental and other conditions, and normalization is a type of psychoeducation (Kingdon & Turkington, 2005). First psychoeducation was used to normalize Rodgerick's culturally specific experience of receiving CBT/mental health treatment for generalized anxiety disorder. Principle 7 (*Critical Evaluation of Clinical and other Relevant Research*) of the RESPPECTUS calls for the critical evaluation and use of research to support CBT with Black clients. Culturally relevant, peer-reviewed research was also used to aid in the normalization of getting help for generalized anxiety disorder and to destigmatize the experience of Rodgerick participating in CBT.

The CBT clinician was aware that Rodgerick may be concerned about receiving CBT if he knew that, relative to White Americans, CBT has been under-researched with individuals in Black samples (Windsor et al., 2015). This fact, compounded with his distrust of systems (as evidenced by his composite scores on the CuTS subscales, Tripartite Police Fear and Beliefs about American and Its Criminal Justice System; see Chap. 5), may be a further deterrent from mental health treatment. The CBT clinician was specifically concerned that Rodgerick may believe that he is being used like "guinea pig" in an outpatient mental health treatment setting. The "guinea pig" phenomenon has been previously cited in research regarding Black mental health treatment research (Williams et al., 2013). The author has seen the same distrust of the mental health systems in outpatient mental health treatment settings as it pertains to psychosocial intervention and pharmacotherapy. After further open-ended questions were used to allow Roderick to express his concerns regarding his role of participating in mental health treatment, Rodgerick was asked by the clinician if the clinician could provide Rodgerick with research regarding the generalized anxiety disorder diagnosis and the CBT treatment. Rodgerick agreed and Rodgerick was informed that anxiety disorders are the most common mental health diagnoses in the United States without respect to race (Bandelow & Michaelis, 2015). As it pertained to treatment without regard to race, Rodgerick was informed that anxiety disorders constituted the second highest diagnoses which received treatment in the United States (Olfson et al., 2019). Rodgerick was informed that for Black Americans anxiety disorders were common (Himle et al., 2009). Research citing the efficacy and promise of CBT with Black Americans diagnosed with generalized anxiety and other disorders was also discussed with Rodgerick (Gregory Jr.,, 2019). The CBT clinician also shared with Rodgerick that he has seen and is seeing other Black individuals in therapy to address other forms of anxiety, fear, and trauma. Rodgerick reported that he appreciated this information as it was helpful for him to know that he was not alone in seeking treatment for anxiety.

6.1.11.2 Alternative Explanation

Rodgerick was first validated for his concerns regarding his decision to participate in therapy and affirmed for the strength it took for him to access therapy. The CBT clinician, being very much aware of various multilevel barriers to Black Americans accessing mental health therapy (Alang, 2019), viewed Rodgerick's being in therapy (despite these barriers) as a strength (principle 1: *Resilience and Strength of Black Americans*). Rodgerick believed that this being in therapy was evidence that he was not good enough. To collaboratively evaluate Rodgerick's thought that he was "not good enough," Rodgerick was asked, "What other ways might you view your being in therapy and addressing anxiety?" (Beck, 2021). Asking Rodgerick this Socratic question presented an opportunity to highlight the strength it took for him to initiate and proceed with the process of getting treatment for anxiety (Principle 1: *Resilience and Strength of Black Americans*). Rodgerick was also asked, "How does you coming to therapy suggest anything positive about you or your decision making?" Rodgerick's responses included the acknowledgment that he was doing something helpful and that his being in therapy was indicative of his positive traits and qualities, which was contrary to the thought that he was not good enough.

6.1.12 Cost-Benefit Analysis: Communal Context, Retrospective, and Prospective

The functional evaluation of thoughts or beliefs embodies the perceived expense and reward of having various cognitions. From a CBT perspective (Beck, 2021), the cost-benefit analysis can have substantive implications for changing emotions and behavior. In CBT, the supposed mechanism by which cost–benefit analysis achieves its effect is based on an objective evaluation that demonstrates the costs of the maladaptive thought or belief are greater than the rewards of having the thought or belief. Conversely, cost–benefit analyses used in motivational interviewing serves the purpose of increasing motivation to change via identifying the discrepancy between one's desired goals and their current state of being (Miller & Rollnick,

2023). The cost–benefit analysis has nuanced components that vary depending on the theoretical framework as well the cultural, historical, and structural context of the clients who use the intervention.

It has been noted that the individualistic nature of CBT could be a barrier to non-White or other cultures (Beck, 2021). However, using principle 1 (*Resilience and Strength of Black Americans*), the predominant collectivist Black culture could be used to further accentuate how the lack of utility for a specific thought could lead to positive emotional and behavioral change. First, a quick review of the collectivist culture in Black Americans is necessary. Black Americans who were enslaved already had a shared communal identity that was developed in West Africa (Jones, 1997). This Black collectivist culture was further developed in response to the traumatic experiences of slavery and resulted in an enhanced shared communal identity based on mutual struggle (Ogbu, 2004). Ogbu maintains that the Black cultural identity developed during slavery is still a prominent factor in determining Black individuals' thoughts about and responses to experiences with White individuals.

For Rodgerick, first, psychoeducation was provided regarding the differences between the life-saving function of fear and the debilitating nature of anxiety (Barlow, 2002). Roderick was then asked to complete the cost–benefit analysis as it pertained to his pro-anxiety thought, "*Anxiety helps protect me from experiencing problems that I worry about*." This thought was categorized as a Mental Filter (Burns, 1989) cognitive distortion, because the supposed benefits were only considered; however, the costs of the thought were neglected. Table 6.1 provides Rodgerick's cost-benefit analysis of his pro-anxiety thought. Rodgerick stated that he thought that his anxiety helped protect him from actually experiencing problems that he worried about. Rodgerick's reported costs of his thoughts were also associated with his reasons for seeking treatment. With regard to the respective benefits and costs of his thought, Rodgerick stated that all things considered, he believed the benefits and costs were more or less equally weighted.

For Black individuals who have a collective Black identity, the costs and benefits of specific thoughts and beliefs could be considered with regard to the historical and prospective collective Black community. One of Rodgerick's strengths was his consistent positive view of both his Black culture and his personal Black identity. Rodgerick had a collective Black identity and a demonstrated understanding of the cognitive model. Therefore, to further examine the utility of Rodgerick's thought, the costs and benefits of his specific, pro-anxiety thought, were considered with regard to the collective Black community. In conducting an Advantage Disadvantage Analysis (similar to a cost–benefit analysis), Liese and Beck (2022) have suggested

Table 6.1 Rodgerick's cost-benefit analysis of his pro-anxiety thought

Benefits of the thought	Costs of the thought
I am more prepared for stressful situations	Feeling physically ill at times, due to worrying
Doing better on exams	Problems relaxing
	Not enjoying life as much
	Lack of control over worrying

Table 6.2 Rodgerick's cost-benefit analysis using his collective Black identity

How did the thought benefit the broader Black community historically?	How could the thought cost the Black community prospectively?
	Historically Black leaders have overcome anxiety to advance progress for all →The cost is the lack of social progress for all
	A pattern of courageous behavior throughout the Black community and Black history resulting in progress for all →The cost is the lack of social progress for all

examining the costs and benefits of a behavior regarding the behavior's effect on important relationships. Similarly, in the cost–benefit analysis with Rodgerick, the costs and benefits of Rodgerick's pro-anxiety thought ("*Anxiety helps protect me from experiencing problems that I worry about.*") was evaluated with regard to how his thought may be reconciled with the history of the broader Black community. With regard to the two columns in Table 6.2, Rodgerick was asked "*How did the thought benefit the broader Black community historically?*" and "*How could the thought costs the Black community prospectively?*"

Rodgerick reported not being able to find any historical benefit of his pro-anxiety thought for the Black community. Rodgerick did find ways in which the thought could negatively impact or cost the Black community prospectively. Specifically, Rodgerick pointed out that Black leaders, in the Black community, have historically overcome fear or anxiety, and the absence of fear or anxiety helped create social progress for the broader society that even extended beyond the Black community. The impact of avoiding behaviors that bring social progress was discussed and analogized with Rodgerick's own avoidance. The discussion included the conflation between highly improbable negative events and the attribution of negative events not occurring, being attributable to anxious thoughts (Norton, 2012). That is, the feared negative events did not occur because of Rodgerick's anxious thoughts that protected him; instead, the feared events did not occur because the likelihood of the feared events occurring was so highly improbable. Rodgerick ultimately concluded that anxiety was not a benefit for the Black community and likely not a benefit for him personally, all things considered (both communal and personal utility of the thought).

6.1.13 Perceived Social Support and Cognitive Intervention with Black Americans

Social support is not routinely viewed in the context of a cognitive intervention. However, perceived social support has been believed by some to be more important than actual social support (Park et al., 2014). The importance of perceived social support, its relationship with cognitive interventions, and its utility for Black people has been seen in psychometric research pertaining to the CuTS. The CuTS's (27 item version, Gregory & Tucker Edmonds, 2024a, Appendix C),

Cognitive-Behavioral Coping Skills subscale, had two items pertaining to perceived community (item 12) and family social support (item 14). These two perceived social support items loaded on the same factor as other items addressing cognitive content (items 15 and 16). In the shortened version of the CuTS (22-item version, Gregory & Tucker Edmonds, 2024b, Appendix D), the perceived social support-oriented items pertaining to friends (item 15), community (item 16), and family (item 17), loaded on the same factor. Due to these items addressing perceptions rather than objective social support and the items previous relationship with other items measuring cognitive content, the perceived social support items were believed to constitute a cognitive-behavioral factor (Gregory & Tucker Edmonds, 2024a, 2024b) and have relevance for cognitive restructuring with Black American men.

The Black American client's perception of social support could be considered a strength (principle 1: *Resilience and Strength of Black Americans*) that may have relevance for cognitive restructuring, depending on the clients CBT case conceptualization. Black clients may have two additional potential sources of perceived social support: extended family and fictive kin (Boyd-Franklin, 2006). According to Boyd-Franklin, extended family (family outside of the family of origin) may offer emotional, financial, and other types of support that are mutually beneficial for both the Black client and the client's extended family. Fictive kin includes supportive/positive individuals with whom the Black client is not biologically related, yet the individuals are referred to and/or treated as being family (Stack, 1983). The author, in his work with Black American clients, has also seen Black individuals who will arrive at a consensus with an extended family member that the family member is considered a family member of origin. The consideration of an extended family member (e.g., a cousin) as a family member of origin (considering the cousin as a little sister or big brother) is based on the perception that the extended family member's relationship and support of the patient have been less like a cousin and more like a family member of origin (a sibling). Kelly (2019) has also previously identified fictive kin as having relevance for CBT.

When Black clients have identified family of origin, extended family, fictive kin, friends, and/or community, these relationships could serve as resources/strengths that further accentuate the Socratic distancing question (Beck, 2021; Leahy, 1996). The distancing question involves the CBT clinician asking the client, what advice would the client give a family member or friend who had the same negative thought or belief? In the case of Rodgerick, he reported having an uncle and cousins (uncle's children) who are more like brothers. Given Rodgerick's thoughts that he is negative and less competent (see *Depression* aspect of initial biopsychosocial assessment), Rodgerick was asked "What feedback would you have for your cousin, if your cousin was having the same negative thoughts?" (Distancing Question, Beck, 2021). Rodgerick reported that he would tell his cousin that he has family, like his father (his cousin's father) and Rodgerick himself, who loves him and supports him and that those thoughts about "not being good enough" are not true. Following Beck's technique, Rodgerick was asked how the same information he applied to his cousin may also apply to him? Rodgerick stated that both he and his cousin have the same family and therefore more or less the same benefits. Rodgerick ultimately acknowledged that the feedback he provided to his cousin does pertain to him; however, sometimes it's hard to see himself positively. Rodgerick correctly identified the thought as Discounting the Positives (Burns, 1989). For homework Roderick was asked to use the Distancing question (D) to respond to his negative thoughts (B) about "not [being] good enough" and less competent. In Chap. 4, the interdependence of the cognitive-behavioral RESPPECTUS principles was described. The aforementioned discussion of the *Evaluating Thoughts and Beliefs* (Principle 6) and *Social Support's Import* (Principle 10) principles illustrate this synergistic quality of the RESPPECTUS principles.

To address the amplified anxiety that typically occurred between the time of the test submission and the test results, Rodgerick was guided in using cognitive and social support strategies that are used during exposures to anxiety-provoking stimuli (Steketee, 1993). One cognitive strategy (principle 6: *Evaluating Thoughts and Beliefs*) was to challenge the thought that he would fail by using the fact that he had had a B average of 3.15 as evidence against the thought that he would fail his test. Between the time of test submission and receipt of the test grade, Rodgerick also agreed to contact his mother and/or uncle to obtain support during the high anxiety time (principle 10: *Social Support's Import*). It should be noted that in his biopsychosocial assessment, Rodgerick perceived some of his professors as being biased against him because he was a Black male. However, for this particular thought, the behavioral experiment did not need to incorporate that aspect of Rodgerick's experience because the focus of attention was Rodgerick's amplified anxiety stemming from his thought, rather than structural racism that created an educational system with biases.

6.1.14 Cognitive Restructuring and the Necessity of Empathy with Black American Clients

Principle 2: *Empathy for Black Traumatic Events and Stressors*, has substantive implications for cognitive restructuring with Black Americans. The importance of empathy has been broadly recognized in CBT principles not specific to Black Americans (Beck, 2021). The importance of empathy is further demonstrated in long-standing clinical research questions regarding whether the active ingredients of CBT or the common factors contribute to therapeutic change (Tolin, 2010). The common factors include those nonmechanistic attributes that are shared among efficacious psychotherapies, for example, therapeutic rapport (Rosenzweig, 1936). While empathy is important for CBT, there is a vast array of racial ideological stances among clinicians that may diminish the empathy expressed in CBT. For example, color-blind racism encompasses beliefs that structural factors are irrelevant to racism, Black culture is inherently responsible for Black disparities, racial issues should not be directly or overtly discussed, and viewing racial disparity as unavoidable and automatic (Bonilla-Silva & Forman, 2000). Research has shown that as clinicians' color-blindness increased, their empathy decreased (Burkard & Knox, 2004).

As it pertains to cultural empathy in CBT, first, the helping professions' historical and structural background regarding racism in psychotherapy must be recognized. Following the public and traumatic homicide of George Floyd in 2020, various professional mental health organizations made public apologies acknowledging the impact of structural and/or other forms of racism stemming from the respective healthcare professions. The American Psychiatric Association (2021), American Psychological Association (2021), and the National Association of Social Workers (2021) issued statements that summarized the respective profession's various roles in contributing to racism of different forms. The question remains: how do CBT clinicians, belonging to various helping professions, adequately convey authentic empathy for Black American clients presenting with racialized stressors, racial trauma, and other mental health issues? After an overview of the roles of empathy for CBT with Black clients, multilevel options for enhancing cultural empathy in CBT are provided.

Empathy has specific functions in CBT with Black American clients:

1. **Conveying Compassion and Respect**: At its most basic level, empathy demonstrates compassion and respect for the Black client, their experience, and world, which contextualizes or even complicates those experiences.
2. **Identification and Sharing of Thoughts/Beliefs**: Empathy for Black Americans participating in CBT is necessary to identify thoughts which are the targets of cognitive interventions. Empathy is paramount in building a therapeutic relationship that facilitates introspection, vulnerability, and transparent sharing of thoughts and beliefs. Some thoughts and beliefs may be associated with racially charged, anti-Black events or experiences. Learning the cognitive model is futile if the therapeutic rapport is not strong enough to facilitate an honest discussion of the Black client's experiences and perceptions of events.
3. **Empathy → Trust → Cognitive Restructuring**: Empathy for Black Americans helps to effectively engage in the cognitive restructuring process. Empathy fosters trust. Trust helps to facilitate a mutual, nonhierarchical partnership in identifying thoughts/beliefs and examining these cognitions for their consistency with reality. Beck (2021) has referred to this process as collaborative empiricism. Expressed empathy from the CBT clinician to the Black client may alleviate or refute some of the client's fears about being heard and understood by a therapist.

What might a CBT clinician do if the clinician wants to effectively convey cultural empathy to a Black client who may be processing issues stemming from structural racism in therapy? Substantive resources exist which provide fundamental concepts regarding empathy (Rogers, 1957) or the methods for creating and sustaining empathy in therapy (Egan & Reese, 2019; Miller & Rollnick, 2023). Clinical social work, psychology, counseling, marriage and family therapy, and other graduate programs typically provide formal coursework on empathy early in the training of clinicians. Workshops or other trainings on therapies that include important components of empathy, including motivational interviewing (engagement; Miller & Rollnick, 2023), and dialectical behavioral therapy (Validation; Linehan, 1993), may have utility for enhancing cultural empathy.

For CBT clinicians, a crucial component of empathy for Black Americans dealing with structural racism is the CBT clinician's own self-awareness of their own beliefs and feelings about anti-Black social injustice. Beck's (1976) acknowledgment that CBT clinicians can impose their own value systems on their clients requires that the CBT clinicians first become aware of their own beliefs and values regarding anti-Black and structural racism. This self-awareness will help detect when the clinician is imposing his own belief system and values on the Black client. There are practitioner and organizational level options for enhancing CBT clinicians' self-awareness of and empathy for anti-Black structural racism. Options for improving clinician empathy in CBT may include training, case staffing with other qualified mental health professionals, individual and/or group clinical supervision, and/or consultation with other clinicians who effectively provide CBT to Black clients. It is also acceptable and preferable for a CBT clinician to decide, in the best interest of the Black client, that he or she is not a suitable candidate to address a client's clinical issues regarding structural racism. It is professionally appropriate not to accept referrals that exceed the CBT clinician's level of expertise and clinical knowledge (Kazantzis et al., 2017). If there is a discrepancy between the agency's staff and the Black client's needs regarding clinical implications of structural racism, it may be helpful to have a network of qualified, empathic CBT clinicians who can receive referrals for such clients. Consulting professional licensing agencies for feedback on appropriate clinical decision making and/or referrals would also be advantageous. When the needs of Black clients are not met by the available clinicians, at the organizational level, it is appropriate to search, screen, recruit, and train those CBT clinicians who are able to competently and compassionately provide CBT with the necessary level of cultural empathy.

6.2 Behavioral Interventions with Black Americans

The first half of this chapter discussed the cognitive model and the application of the RESPPECTUS principles to cognitive interventions with Black American clients. The second half of this chapter focuses on behavioral interventions with Black American clients and the role of the RESPPECTUS principles in augmenting these interventions. Behavioral interventions are relevant for several reasons. The source of the Black client's problems does not always stem from the client's distorted thoughts or beliefs. The problem causing distress in the Black client's life may be largely environmental or have both intrapersonal and environmental components. Linehan (1993), discussing the use of cognitive restructuring with clients who have borderline disorder, pointed out that these clients are frequently told that their thoughts and beliefs are distorted. Similarly, Black individuals within American are frequently invalidated for their perceptions of anti-Black racism and discrimination in America (Yi et al., 2022). Given structural, historical, and contemporary racism, behavioral interventions can be used as skills to effectively respond to anti-Black racism and discrimination as well as symptoms associated with the Black client's diagnoses. If indeed the Black client's issue is cognitive in nature, behavioral interventions may also be a mechanism to change maladaptive thoughts and beliefs (Norton, 2012). The behavioral interventions presented in this chapter primarily are in the category of skill building (Farmer & Chapman, 2008) because these interventions are intended to be used for addressing symptoms of mental illness and racial stressors. The behavioral interventions also serve the role of building on already existing skill sets and resources that each Black client brings to therapy (principle 1: *Resilience and Strength of Black Americans*).

6.2.1 Problem-Solving

Problem-solving is considered a principle by itself (principle 5: *Problem-Solving*) because of the intervention's great utility for Black American issues that are environmental in nature. Problem-solving involves a series of steps (D'Zurilla & Nezu, 1999):

1. Defining the problem.
2. Defining the goal(s).
3. Identifying potential solutions to the problem.
4. Choosing one or more solutions.
5. Implementing the solution(s).
6. Evaluating the outcomes.

Using the case of Rodgerick, each of the problem-solving steps was followed while incorporating several of the RESPPECTUS principles. A rationale for the problem-solving model was provided to Rodgerick. The rationale for the problem-solving model was provided by distinguishing the problem-solving model from the cognitive model. The cognitive model was summarized as using cognitive interventions to evaluate and potentially replace thoughts which may negatively influence Rodgerick's mood and behavior. The problem-solving model, to the contrary was used to resolve problems that do not stem from Rodgerick's thoughts but are based in Rodgerick's environment or interpersonal situations. Rodgerick's use of the problem-solving model was applied to a situation regarding a grade that Rodgerick believed was not indicative of his work. Rodgerick had reported that some of his worry comes from his grades that he received and may get in the future. Recall that Rodgerick believed that he has been given lower grades than his actual work indicated because of his professor's perceptions of the academic performance of Black males. Rodgerick described a situation with his history professor and his receiving a C grade on his exam. Rodgerick's application of the problem-solving model (D'Zurilla & Nezu, 1999), while incorporating the RESPPECTUS principles is listed as follows:

1. *Defining the Problem*: Rodgerick discussed his believing that he was unfairly judged and graded by several of his college professors. Rodgerick's definition of the problem included his receiving a C on a history exam that he believed he should have got at least a B on.
2. *Defining the Goal*: Rodgerick reports that he wanted to at least receive a B on his exam, as he believed that this was indeed the grade that he earned. Rodgerick reported that he wanted the professor to change his grade.
3. *Identifying Potential Solutions to the Problem*:
   a. Doing nothing and hoping for the best.
   b. Getting feedback from his uncle on how to resolve the issue.
   c. Giving his professor a bad evaluation at the end of the semester.
   d. Speaking to his professor regarding the grade he received on his exam and advocating for why he believes he should have received a better grade.
   e. Using this experience to learn what he might do differently on exams in the future.
4. *Choosing One or More Solutions*:
   a. After evaluating the potential pros and cons of each solution, Rodgerick decided that he was going to email the professor and ask to meet with him regarding his concerns about how his exam was graded and that he would use this as a learning experience for this and future courses.
5. *Implementing the Solution(s)*:
   a. Rodgerick met with his professor after class and discussed his concerns regarding the grade. Rodgerick discussed his perceived discrepancy between his response to the question and the grade he received.
6. *Evaluating the Outcomes*:
   a. Rodgerick reported that his professor understood his point of view and believed his concerns had merit. Rodgerick reported that the change to his grade on that particular response resulted in him getting a B- on the exam.

The CBT clinician was aware of structural racism's impact on educational outcomes (principle 3: *Structural Racism*) pertaining to Black males in America. The clinician believed that Rodgerick claims were generally supported by both historical and contemporary race and gender bias issues within the American educational system (Banaji et al., 2021). Beck (1976) maintained that a thought is considered maladaptive if the CBT clinician and client agree that the cognition hinders the client's progress or goals. Therefore, the CBT clinician also did not use a cognitive intervention regarding Rodgerick's belief (that his professor had judged him based on his race and gender) because Rodgerick had already concluded that the grade was inappropriate and was a result of intersecting race and gender bias from the professor. The CBT clinician also considered the potential impact of evaluating Rodgerick's belief on his therapeutic rapport with Rodgerick. The clinician believed that attempting to evaluate the belief, given all the considered factors, would damage his rapport with the client (Principle 2: *Empathy for Black Traumatic Events and Stressors*).

In working with Rodgerick on the problem-solving model, Rodgerick was asked "What strengths or positive things, could you use to help resolve this problem?" Rodgerick reported that he studied and knew the material on the exam, could talk to his uncle and seek his uncle's advice on the problem, has been present for all of the course lectures—never missed a class, and reports that his response on the exam was factually correct. When asked for any other strengths which may be present, Rodgerick stated that he has a history of being successful in school, although he has never been a straight A student. While Rodgerick did not receive the B that he believed he had earned Rodgerick reported that he learned more about himself by working through the problem-solving model to address the issue. Working through the problem-solving model demonstrated some evidence to the contrary of his low self-efficacy and other negative thoughts about himself. The problem-solving intervention not only was a demonstration of how a skill could be used to address an issue, the action-oriented aspects of the problem-solving model also provided Rodgerick with an opportunity to disconfirm some of the anxious and depressive thoughts that he had about himself.

6.2.2 Behavioral Experiment

Behavioral experiments are based on the premise that cognitions can be supported or disconfirmed through evidence that is obtained from planned tasks that serve as experiments (Farmer & Chapman, 2008). Behavioral experiments can be beneficial for individuals, such as Rodgerick, with low self-efficacy (Bandura, 1986). Rodgerick reported low self-efficacy regarding his ability to cope with anxiety and disruptive worrying associated with his submitted assignments. Rodgerick's thoughts typically involved the notion that he was going to fail his exams after submitting them. This thought pertaining to Rodgerick's exams represented Emotional Reasoning (Burns, 1989) because Rodgerick's anxious mood was the source of his pessimistic thoughts regarding his exams.

Rodgerick collaborated with his CBT clinician regarding a behavioral experiment that could be used to test his defeatist thoughts about the negative outcomes of his submitted exams. Rodgerick was guided in conducting an experiment to test his thought that he would fail his exams. The rationale for behavioral experiments was discussed with Rodgerick. Rodgerick provided an operational definition for what "fail" meant. Rogerick's definition of failure was anything less than a C-. Rodgerick stated that if he studied for exams, while trying to reduce his worrying and got scores greater than a C-, "that would suggest worrying is not helpful or justified for the most part" (alternative thought). Rodgerick stated that he had an exam in his sociology course, and this would be an opportunity to conduct the behavioral experiment. Rodgerick's experiment first included setting aside a specific time and making a plan to study for the sociology exam. Rodgerick stated that studying his book and notes from the professor's class were the best methods to prepare for the exam. Rodgerick took the exam and awaited the score. Rodgerick received a B and therefore concluded that this initial behavioral experiment supported his alternative thought.

6.3 Cognitive-Behavioral Therapy and Homework with Black Americans

Homework is a key component of CBT; homework allows clients time to practice cognitive-behavioral skills (learned in session) in a real-world environment (Kazantzis, 2005). Research has suggested that homework between sessions can be optimized by the following (Ryum et al., 2023):

- Working with the client to co-design the homework assignment.
- Ensuring that the homework assignment is linked to the content of the session.
- Providing a comprehensive rationale for the homework assignment.
- Talking about the potential obstacles to completing the homework assignment with the client.
- Providing the homework assignment in writing.
- Listening to and taking client feedback into consideration.
- Incorporating the client's environmental circumstances into the homework assignment.

Similar to Ryum and associates, when discussing the need to make sociocultural adaptations for homework, Tompkins (2004) makes a number of recommendations. Tompkins states the importance of making sure the homework assignment is within the client's capability to complete. For example, the homework assignment should be compatible with the client's financial capability. Tompkins also suggests making sure the client perceives the homework assignment as being clearly related to their problem. Seeking feedback from professionals with culture-specific knowledge and working with family members of the client regarding ways to improve completion of homework is also suggested by Tompkins. Recall that Black Americans, fictive kin and extended family (Boyd-Franklin, 2006) were discussed in this chapter as it pertains to social support. Tompkins recommends that clinicians work with these additional family members to increase the likelihood that homework will be completed.

In the author's own work with Black Americans, developing homework assignments using CBT, the term that is used to specify the "homework" or between-session exercise is important and may contribute to or decrease the likelihood that the homework is completed. Again, in the authors on work with Black Americans, the term "homework" to describe between-session exercises was often not preferred. The author has found, for some of Black American clients he has worked with, the term homework often invoked hierarchical or adversarial relationships stemming from past negative educational experiences. Instead, the author would use the term "practice" or "exercises." Consistent with principle 9 (*Uniqueness of Each Black Individual*), no one term will always be preferred by all Black Americans. Each cognitive-behavioral clinician will need to engage and work with the Black client to determine the best term to use when referring to between-session homework assignments.

6.4 Cognitive-Behavioral Interventions—Integrating RESPPECTUS Principles: Summary

In this chapter, Black American relevant use of cognitive and behavioral interventions was discussed in the context of the cognitive-behavioral RESPPECTUS principles. Cognitive restructuring and behavioral interventions for Black clients, with examples from the case of Rodgerick, were provided. Throughout the discussion of cognitive restructuring, specific RESPPECTUS principles were referenced: *Resilience and Strength of Black Americans* (principle 1), *Empathy for Black Traumatic Events and Stressors* (principle 2), *Structural Racism* (principle 3), *Policy Change* (principle 5), *Evaluating Thoughts and Beliefs* (principle 6), *Critical Evaluation of Clinical and other Relevant Research* (principle 7), *Uniqueness of Each Black Individual* (principle 9), and *Social Support's Import* (principle 10).

The use of the RESPPECTUS principles for behavioral intervention with Black Americans receiving CBT was discussed and applied to the case of Rodgerick. It is important to note that the RESPPECTUS principles were tailored to the unique strengths and resources which Rodgerick had available. Rodgerick had social support that could be leveraged to aid him in achieving his goals. Other clients may be more racially isolated, not have readily available social support, and/or may require additional behavioral skill building such as assertiveness or communication skills. Depending on the Black American client, the way in which the RESPPECTUS principles are applied may vary depending on the client's initial assessment, cognitive-behavioral conceptualization, the client's preferences, and other factors. For example, the Christian religion and spirituality had some overlap with cognitive-behavioral interventions, and this was suitable for Rodgerick given his religious and spiritual beliefs and values. However, research has also shown that some Black Americans view their religious beliefs as being incongruent with therapy (Ayalon & Alvidrez, 2007). Other Black American clients may belong to a different religion or a different Christian denomination that may have specific beliefs and practices that have implications for the CBT case conceptualization and subsequent cognitive-behavioral interventions. The next chapter (Chap. 7) discusses the use of cognitive-behavioral group therapy with Black Americans and applies the RESPPECTUS principles to that treatment modality.

References

Alang, S. M. (2019). Mental health care among blacks in America: Confronting racism and constructing solutions. *Health Services Research, 54*(2), 346–355. https://doi.org/10.1111/1475-6773.13115

Alford, B. A., & Beck, A. T. (1997). *The integrative power of cognitive therapy*. Guilford Press.

American Psychiatric Association. (2021, January 18). *APA's apology to Black, indigenous and people of color for its support of structural racism in psychiatry*. https://www.psychiatry.org/news-room/apa-apology-for-its-support-of-structural-racism

American Psychological Association. (2021, October). *Apology to people of color for APA's role in promoting, perpetuating, and failing to challenge racism, racial discrimination, and human hierarchy in U.S. Resolution adopted by the APA council of representatives on October 29, 2021*. https://www.apa.org/about/policy/racism-apology

Ayalon, L., & Alvidrez, J. (2007). The experience of black consumers in the mental health system--identifying barriers to and facilitators of mental health treatment using the consumers' perspective. *Issues in Mental Health Nursing, 28*(12), 1323–1340. https://doi.org/10.1080/01612840701651454

Banaji, M. R., Fiske, S. T., & Massey, D. S. (2021). Systemic racism: Individuals and interactions, institutions and society. *Cognitive Research: Principles and Implications, 6*, 82. https://doi.org/10.1186/s41235-021-00349-3

Bandelow, B., & Michaelis, S. (2015). Epidemiology of anxiety disorders in the 21st century. *Dialogues in Clinical Neuroscience, 17*(3), 327–335. https://doi.org/10.31887/DCNS.2015.17.3/bbandelow

Bandura, A. (1986). *Social foundations of thought and action: A social cognitive theory*. Prentice-Hall.

Barlow, D. H. (2002). *Anxiety and its disorders: The nature and treatment of anxiety and panic*. Guilford Press.

Beck, A. T. (1976). *Cognitive therapy and the emotional disorders*. Meridian.

Beck, J. S. (2021). *Cognitive behavior therapy: Basics and beyond* (3rd ed.). Guilford Press.

Beck, A. T., Rush, A. J., Shaw, B. F., & Emery, G. (1979). *Cognitive therapy of depression*. Guilford Press.

Beck, A. T., Wright, F. D., Newman, C. F., & Liese, B. S. (1993). *Cognitive therapy of substance abuse*. Guilford Press.

Berger, P. L., & Luckmann, T. (1966). *The social construction of reality: A treatise in the sociology of knowledge*. Anchor Books.

Bishop, F. M. (2001). *Managing addictions: Cognitive, emotive, and behavioral techniques*. Jason Aronson.

Bonilla-Silva, E., & Forman, T. A. (2000). "I am not a racist but ...": mapping White college students' racial ideology in the USA. *Discourse and Society, 11*(1), 50–85. https://doi.org/10.1177/0957926500011001003

Boyd-Franklin, N. (2006). *Black families in therapy A multisystems approach* (2nd ed.). Guilford Press.

Burkard, A. W., & Knox, S. (2004). Effect of therapist color-blindness on empathy and attributions in cross-cultural counseling. *Journal of Counseling Psychology, 51*(4), 387–397.

Burns, D. D. (1989). *The feeling good handbook*. Penguin Books.

Carroll, K. M. (1998). *A cognitive-behavioral approach: Treating cocaine addiction*. National Institute on Drug Abuse.

D'Zurilla, J. J., & Nezu, A. M. (1999). *Problem-solving therapy: A social competence approach to clinical intervention* (2nd ed.). Springer Publications Company.

Dobson, K. S. (2012). *Cognitive therapy*. American Psychological Association.

Edberg, M. (2022). *Essentials of health, culture, and diversity: Understanding people, reducing disparities* (2nd ed.).

Egan, G., & Reese, R. J. (2019). *The skilled helper: A problem-management & opportunity-development approach to helping* (11th ed.). Cengage.

Ellis, A. (1994). *Reason and emotion in psychotherapy: A comprehensive method of treating human disturbances*.(Revised and updated. Carol Publishing Group.

Farmer, R. F., & Chapman, A. L. (2008). *Behavioral interventions in cognitive behavior therapy: Practical guidance for putting theory into action*. American Psychological Association.

Goode-Cross, D. T., & Grim, K. A. (2016). "An unspoken level of comfort": Black therapists' experiences working with Black clients. *Journal of Black Psychology, 42*(1), 29–53. https://doi.org/10.1177/0095798414552103

Gordon, C. D. (2023). Just What Is Afropessimism and What's It Doing in a Nice Field Like Education?: Unpacking New Contributions to Black Educational Thought. *Race, Ethnicity and Education, 26*(1), 18–33. https://doi.org/10.1080/13613324.2022.2122522

Gregory, V. L., Jr. (2019). Cognitive-behavioral therapy for anxious symptoms in persons of African descent: A meta-analysis. *Journal of Social Service Research, 45*(1), 87–101. https://doi.org/10.1080/01488376.2018.1479344

Gregory, V. L., Jr., & Clary, K. L. (2022). Addressing anti-Black racism: The roles of social work. *Smith College Studies in Social Work, 92*(1), 1–27. https://doi.org/10.1080/00377317.2021.2008287

Gregory, V. L., Jr., & Tucker Edmonds, J. L. (2023). The racial pandemic experienced by Black American men: Cognitive-behavioral and structural implications. *American Journal of Orthopsychiatry, 93*(1), 1–16. https://doi.org/10.1037/ort0000651

Gregory, V. L., Jr., & Tucker Edmonds, J. L. (2024a). Cultural Trauma Scale: Psychometric evaluation of Black men's beliefs, emotions, and coping. *Psychological Trauma: Theory, Research, Practice, and Policy, 16*(8), 1329–1337. https://doi.org/10.1037/tra0001607

Gregory, V. L., Jr., & Tucker Edmonds, J. L. (2024b). Cultural Trauma Scale (CuTS): Parsimonious principal component analysis, independent Black American male sample. *Journal of Aggression, Maltreatment and Trauma, 33*(3), 369–386. https://doi.org/10.1080/10926771.2023.2256741

Gregory, V. L., Jr., Miller, B. L., & Lipsey, A. (in press). Black men, structural racism, cultural barriers: Structural equation model with cognitive-behavioral implications. *The Counseling Psychologist.*

Gregory, V. L., Jr., Zapolski, T., Marriott, B. R., Lipsey, A., Hicks, A. I., & Lee, C. (2025). *Exploring the lived experience of Black Americans and substance use treatment: Structural, community, and individual factors*. [Manuscript submitted]. School of Social Work, Indiana University.

Himle, J. A., Baser, R. E., Taylor, R. J., Campbell, R. D., & Jackson, J. S. (2009). Anxiety disorders among African Americans, blacks of Caribbean descent, and non-Hispanic whites in the United States. *Journal of anxiety disorders, 23*(5), 578–590. https://doi.org/10.1016/j.janxdis.2009.01.002

Joe, J. R., Shillingford-Butler, M. A., & Oh, S. (2019). The experiences of African American mothers raising sons in the context of #BlackLivesMatter. *The Professional Counselor, 9*(1), 67–79. https://doi.org/10.15241/jrj.9.1.67

Jones, R. (1997). Individualism: Eighteenth century origins—twentieth century consequences. *The Western Journal of Black Studies, 21*(1), 20–33.

Kazantzis, N. (2005). Introduction and overview. In N. Kazantzis, F. P. Deane, K. R. Ronan, & L. L'Abate (Eds.), *Using homework assignments in cognitive behavior therapy* (pp. 1–6). Routeledge.

Kazantzis, N., Dattilio, F. M., & Dobson, K. S. (2017). *The therapeutic relationship in cognitive-behavioral therapy: A clinician's guide*. Guilford Press.

Kelly, S. (2019). Cognitive behavior therapy with African Americans. In G. Y. Iwamasa & P. A. Hays (Eds.), *Culturally responsive cognitive behavior therapy: Practice and supervision* (2nd ed., pp. 105–128). American Psychological Association. https://doi.org/10.1037/0000119-005

Kingdon, D. G., & Turkington, D. (2005). *Cognitive therapy of schizophrenia*. Guilford Press.

Kugelmass, H. (2016). 'Sorry, I'm not accepting new patients': An audit study of access to mental health care. *Journal of Health and Social Behavior, 57*(2), 168–183. https://doi.org/10.1177/0022146516647098

Leahy, R. (1996). *Cognitive therapy: Basic principles and applications*. Jason Aronson.

Liese, B. S., & Beck, A. T. (2022). *Cognitive-behavioral therapy of addictive disorders*. Guilford Press.

Linehan, J. M. (1993). *Cognitive-behavioral treatment of borderline personality disorder*. The Guilford Press.

Marlatt, G. A. (1985). The cognitive factors in the relapse process. In G. A. Marlatt & J. R. Gordon (Eds.), *Relapse prevention* (pp. 128–200). Guilford Press.

Miller, W. R., & Rollnick, S. (2023). *Motivational interviewing: Helping people change and grow* (4th ed.). Guilford Press.

National Association of Social Workers. (2021, June 17). *NASW apologizes for racist practices in American social work*. https://www.socialworkers.org/LinkClick.aspx?fileticket=29AYH9qAdXc%3d&portalid=0

New International Version Holy Bible. (2011). Zondervan.

Norton, P. J. (2012). *Group cognitive-behavioral therapy of anxiety: A transdiagnostic treatment manual.* .

Ogbu, J. U. (2004). Collective identity and the burden of "Acting White" in Black History, Community, and Education. *Urban Review, 36*(1), 1–35. https://doi.org/10.1023/B:URRE.0000042734.83194.f6

Olfson, M., Blanco, C., Wall, M. M., Liu, S. M., & Grant, B. F. (2019). Treatment of common mental disorders in the United States: Results from the national epidemiologic survey on alcohol and related conditions-III. *The Journal of Clinical Psychiatry, 80*(3), 18m12532. https://doi.org/10.4088/JCP.18m12532

Park, M., Cuijpers, P., Straten, A., & Reynolds, C. (2014). The effects of psychotherapy for adult depression on social support: A meta-analysis. *Cognitive Therapy and Research, 38*(6), 600–611. https://doi.org/10.1007/s10608-014-9630-z

Pew Research Center. (2021, February 16). *Faith among Black Americans*. https://www.pewresearch.org/religion/2021/02/16/faith-among-black-americans/

Pyke, K. D. (2010). What is internalized racial oppression and why don't we study it? Acknowledging racism's hidden injuries. *Sociological Perspectives, 53*(4), 551–572. https://doi.org/10.1525/sop.2010.53.4.551

Rogers, C. R. (1957). The necessary and sufficient conditions of therapeutic personality change. *Journal of Consulting Psychology, 21*(2), 95–103. https://doi.org/10.1037/h0045357

Rosenzweig, S. (1936). Some implicit common factors in diverse methods of psychotherapy. *American Journal of Orthopsychiatry, 6*(3), 412–415. https://doi.org/10.1111/j.1939-0025.1936.tb05248.x

Ryum, T., Bennion, M., & Kazantzis, N. (2023). Integrating between-session homework in psychotherapy: A systematic review of immediate in-session and intermediate outcomes. *Psychotherapy, 60*(3), 306–319. https://doi.org/10.1037/pst0000488

Scott, L. D., Jr., & Davis, L. E. (2006). Young, black, and male in foster care: Relationship of negative social contextual experiences to factors relevant to mental health service delivery. *Journal of Adolescence, 29*(5), 721–736. https://doi.org/10.1016/j.adolescence.2005.11.002

Smith, T. B., & Silva, L. (2011). Ethnic Identity and Personal Well-Being of People of Color: A Meta-Analysis. *Journal of Counseling Psychology, 58*(1), 42–60. https://doi.org/10.1037/a0021528

Stack, C. (1983). *All our kin: Strategies for survival in a Black community*. Basic Books.

Steketee, G. S. (1993). *Treatment of obsessive-compulsive disorder*. Guilford Press.

Tolin, D. F. (2010). Is cognitive-behavioral therapy more effective than other therapies? A meta-analytic review. *Clinical Psychology Review, 30*(6), 710–720. https://doi.org/10.1016/j.cpr.2010.05.003

Tompkins, M. A. (2004). *Using homework in psychotherapy: Strategies, guidelines, and forms.* Guilford Press.

Turner, E. A., Harrell, S. P., & Bryant-Davis, T. (2022). Black Love, Activism, and Community (BLAC): The BLAC model of healing and resilience. *Journal of Black Psychology, 48*(3/4), 547–568. https://doi.org/10.1177/00957984211018364

Williams, M. T., Beckmann-Mendez, D. A., & Turkheimer, E. (2013). Cultural barriers to African American participation in anxiety disorders research. *Journal of the National Medical Association, 105*(1), 33–41. https://doi.org/10.1016/s0027-9684(15)30083-3

Windsor, L. C., Jemal, A., & Alessi, E. J. (2015). Cognitive behavioral therapy: A meta-analysis of race and substance use outcomes. *Cultural Diversity and Ethnic Minority Psychology, 21*(2), 300–313. https://doi.org/10.1037/a0037929

Yi, J., Neville, H. A., Todd, N. R., & Mekawi, Y. (2022). Ignoring race and denying racism: A meta-analysis of the associations between colorblind racial ideology, anti-blackness, and other variables antithetical to racial justice. *Journal of Counseling Psychology, 70*(3), 258–275. https://doi.org/10.1037/cou0000618

Chapter 7
Cognitive-Behavioral Group Therapy: Integrating RESPPECTUS Principles

7.1 Structural Racism and Group Therapy

How does structural racism influence group therapy? Groups are influenced by and indicative of broader micro and macro social realities (Yalom & Leszcz, 2020). One impact of structural racism on group therapy is the manifestations of microaggressive anti-Black behaviors. Microaggressions are subtle forms of discrimination (Pierce et al., 1977). Racial microaggressions have been significantly and positively correlated with adjustment problems, especially for internalizing symptoms and stress (Lui & Quezada, 2019). Research has shown that microaggressions in group therapy occur at a high rate (Kivlighan III et al., 2021). Groups have been referred to as intricate, multitiered, and potentially requiring a multitiered approach to resolve microaggressive behavior (Miles et al., 2021). Before considering how the RESPPECTUS principles may be used to decrease microaggressive behavior regarding Black American clients, first more broader considerations of cognitive-behavioral group therapy, the efficacy of cognitive-behavioral group therapy, and Yalom's therapeutic factors (Yalom & Leszcz, 2020) with Black Americans are discussed.

7.2 Cognitive-Behavioral Group Therapy and Black Americans

Cognitive-behavioral group therapy capitalizes on the synergy among cognitive-behavioral theory, cognitive-behavioral interventions, and positive aspects of the therapeutic group dynamic. Cognitive-behavioral group therapy has been used to treat a variety of DSM disorders, including but not limited to schizophrenia, substance-related, anxiety, personality, and depressive disorders (Bieling et al., 2022). Similar to individual cognitive-behavioral therapy (CBT),

V. L. Gregory, Jr., *Cognitive-Behavioral Therapy with Black Americans*,
https://doi.org/10.1007/978-3-032-01666-9_7

cognitive-behavioral group therapy also has key cognitive-behavioral features, such as structure, as well as cognitive and behavioral interventions that are enhanced by the group format. The seminal text on group therapy is Yalom's *The Theory and Practice of Group Therapy* (Yalom & Leszcz, 2020). The text highlights some of the powerful components of group therapy. Yalom has referred to these beneficial components of group therapy as therapeutic factors. The frequently cited therapeutic factors of group therapy include (Yalom & Leszcz, 2020): hope, mutual support, shared experiences, educational components, social skills, cohesiveness, and modeling of positive behaviors, among others. Bieling et al. (2022) have discussed the ways in which group CBT advances many of Yalom's therapeutic factors. For example, cognitive-behavioral groups on specific disorders enhance the universality and may decrease stigma among individuals who share the same disorder. Group feedback on cognitive restructuring exercises adds to the group's altruism. Bieling and associates also discuss how group therapy could be used to advance the behavioral coping skills of CBT (Yalom's socializing and imitative behavior therapeutic factors).

Cognitive-behavioral group therapy for Black Americans can occur in several forms. There are CBT groups which are specifically constructed solely for Black individuals to address mental health or other psychosocial problems and their Black cultural nexus. Take, for example, the culturally adapted cognitive-behavioral group intervention by Webb Hooper and associates (2017), which was focused on nicotine cessation for Black Americans with lower SES. There are also racially heterogenous groups that address different mental health problems, whom Black individuals are a part of. The use of cognitive-behavioral group therapy focused solely on Black individuals and Black individuals in racially heterogenous groups is likely determined by the cultural context of the treatment, the geographic location and the racial makeup of the treatment location, the mission of the agency, and the skill set of the providers.

7.3 Cognitive-Behavioral Group Therapy: Clinical Trials with Black Americans

Systematic reviews and clinical trials have examined the use of culturally adapted cognitive-behavioral group therapy for Black Americans. Similar to other CBT clinical trials with Black Americans, the empirical research is relatively limited, yet promising. A vote counting systematic review by Kunorubwe (2023) reviewed culturally adapted cognitive-behavioral group therapy for racially diverse clients with depression. The systematic review showed that 9 of the 10 studies had statistically significant findings that favored cognitive-behavioral group therapy. However, similar to other cognitive-behavioral systematic review research that was previously discussed in Chap. 1, the study by Kunorubwe was limited because it did not focus exclusively on Black Americans, and it did not aggregate effect sizes. The clinical trials that included Black Americans in this systematic review were found to have statistically significant findings that favored cognitive-behavioral group therapy (Bowe, 2013; Ward & Brown, 2015) or had findings with a direction that favored cognitive-behavioral group therapy (Kohn et al., 2002). An randomized controlled trial examined the efficacy of cognitive-behavioral group therapy for Black American women with panic disorder (Carter et al., 2003). The results favored cognitive-behavioral group therapy, relative to the control, and had a large effect size in reducing anxiety. Another study (Ali, 2008) used a pretest–posttest design in a cognitive-behavioral marathon group intervention with Black women that had human immunodeficiency virus (HIV). The study had a moderate effect size and favored the CBT intervention in the reduction of anxiety.

With the positive outcomes seen in the aforementioned clinical trials, it begs the question of what mechanism of cognitive-behavioral group therapy may be associated with improvement? The author and several associates conducted a qualitative study with Black individuals who had experienced substance use treatment (Gregory Jr. et al., 2025). One of the many important findings was the experience of Yalom's therapeutic factors (Yalom & Leszcz, 2020) among Black individuals who participated in group therapy sessions. Over a fourth of the participants alluded to experiencing Yalom's therapeutic factors in group therapy: instillation of hope, imparting information, altruism, catharsis, universality, and cohesiveness.

7.4 Yalom's Therapeutic Factors and Black Cognitive-Behavioral Group Therapy Participants

Cognitive-behavioral therapy and group therapy are synergistic and complementary. The addition of Black participants in cognitive-behavioral group therapy has the potential to amplify the clinical and cultural benefits of cognitive-behavioral group therapy involving Black American participants. Below are each of Yalom's therapeutic factors (Yalom & Leszcz, 2020) discussed in relation to how the specific characteristics can be advanced by Black Americans participating in cognitive-behavioral group therapy.

Hope may be increased in group therapy via a number of factors; a group member seeing other group members improve, a group member being validated by the clinician for progress the group member has made, or a group member's belief that the therapy is working (Yalom & Leszcz, 2020). With Black Americans in cognitive-behavioral group therapy, hope may be facilitated via watching another group member consider evidence to the contrary of a maladaptive thought. The author has conducted cognitive restructuring exercises in group therapy, where one Black group member has a maladaptive thought that is similar to another Black group member's maladaptive manner of thinking. When one Black group member identifies substantive evidence that counteracts the negative thought, other Black group members may positively consider the extent to which that same evidence contradicts their own negative and maladaptive thinking. This process not only facilitates cognitive restructuring, but it may also fuel hope. When Black Americans hear their White counterparts overcoming various struggles in group therapy, the Black participant may ask themselves how the same success could be achieved for themselves, given anti-Black structural racism which pervades every aspect of American society. Although it must be stated and in accordance with principle 9, *Uniqueness of Each Black Individual*, many and certainly not all Black individuals will have this question. The development of hope may occur when Black clients hear and see how other Black Americans triumph over racism and discrimination. This capacity for Black individuals to catalyze hope in one another, within cognitive-behavioral group therapy settings, can synergize the benefits of cognitive-behavioral group therapy with Black Americans.

Universality refers to the awareness a client in groups has when the group member learns that other group members have experiences that are similar to theirs (Yalom & Leszcz, 2020). The concept of universality can be advanced among Black cognitive-behavioral group therapy participants by Black Americans hearing other Black individuals share their experiences, thoughts, and feelings regarding their strengths, resilience, and experiences with mental illness, racism, and discrimination. In a social environment where Black individuals are often invalidated for discussing the experiences or impact of racism (empathic isolation; Joe et al., 2019), Black Americans in group therapy may receive validation from other Black individuals who struggle with and overcome some of the same racial discrimination. The concept of universality in group therapy may also challenge attribution errors of Black individuals who may disproportionately attribute fault or blame to themselves (personalization and blame cognitive distortion; Burns, 1989).

In group therapy, imparting information includes beneficial information coming from both the clinician and other group members (Yalom & Leszcz, 2020). When Black individuals are present in the same cognitive-behavioral group therapy sessions, information may be shared among the Black group members that is indicative of the Black culture. The potential drawback of being the only Black member in a cognitive-behavioral group therapy session is that, while other non-Black group members may be well-intentioned, feedback may be provided that is not consistent with the cultural or socially constructed reality of the Black individual's community. Having Black members in a group therapy session may potentially increase the likelihood of information being provided that is culturally relevant and therefore more likely to be useful. However, it must also be stated that having a cognitive-behavioral group therapy session with members of different races may also be beneficial because Black group members may potentially get different perspectives or hear a perspective that the individual does not usually hear. The impartation of information, be it from Black or non-Black group members, may potentially provide an alternative perspective that is contrary to a negative thought that facilitates undesirable emotions and behaviors. The author has conducted group therapy sessions where Black individuals have shared culturally relevant information that consisted of resources to resolve practical problems that were disproportionately experienced by Black individuals due to social and healthcare disparities. For example, this sharing of information sometimes consisted of good healthcare providers who were respectful of and sensitive to the needs of Black individuals or community resources that could help with socioeconomic concerns that a Black individual experienced in a group.

Altruism is beneficial in group therapy because group members help one another and receive a benefit from helping another person and from receiving help (Yalom & Leszcz, 2020). Race may play an important role in group therapy because some Black individuals may enter group therapy somewhat reluctantly, preferring individual therapy rather than a group modality due to anticipated racial concerns and past negative experiences. While altruism may be present in a group therapy session that is predominantly White, some Black individuals may be less willing to access the supports of group therapy due to an acknowledged or unacknowledged lack of trust for other members of the group. This may be especially true when a Black individual newly begins attending predominantly White group therapy sessions. In situations where the Black individual has a positive racial identity and is looking to connect with other Black individuals, the presence of other Black individuals in a group session may provide some basic support for trust and altruism to be experienced by Black individuals within a group therapy session. Alternatively, Black individuals receiving support from other non-Black group therapy participants may serve to disconfirm any potential negative thoughts and ultimately build trust that may translate to social experiences outside of group therapy.

The group therapy session may in many ways mimic the structure and context of a family (Yalom & Leszcz, 2020). The group therapy session provides a unique situation for the Black American concepts of fictive kin (Stack, 1983) and extended family (Boyd-Franklin, 1991) to be effectively utilized. The concepts of fictive kin and extended family collectively speak to a shared sense of unity that centers Blackness (culture), shared Black experiences, and transcends various forms of Black division. In multiracial cognitive-behavioral group therapy sessions, this shared sense of Black unity may, at least in theory, aid in engagement as Black participants may feel some sense of shared identity and belonging by seeing other Black individuals. The author frequently worked in group therapy sessions, and depending on the week, the racial makeup of the group could have been anywhere from 10% to 90% Black group therapy members. In groups that were largely multiracial, similar to families (Nichols & Davis, 2017), the author would observe subsystems within the group, where Black individuals would become a subgroup based on their shared experiences around the clinical group content and their shared experiences in life overall. This Black subgroup, within the racially heterogenous therapy group, may have provided a subsystem of support where Black group members may have otherwise believed they were estranged from the group based on a lack of racial connection with the other non-Black group members.

Yalom and Leszcz (2020) have discussed how group participants will sometimes respond to group facilitators the same way that the group participants responded to their parents. The author has conducted youth groups, and the author has on occasion noticed that some Black male teenagers who had tumultuous or strained relationships with their Black fathers would view the Black male author (who was the

Black group member's group therapist) in the same negative light. When this occurred, as the therapist, the author was able to document this father-child strained relationship in the cognitive-behavioral case conceptualization and theorize how the young Black male's experience with his own father may have shaped the Black male group member's beliefs about the author/therapist. These issues were important to consider as they pertained to the therapeutic rapport with that specific young Black male group therapy member and the overall group therapeutic rapport.

Yalom has pointed out that group therapy provides a resource for the explicit and implicit provision of social skills (Yalom & Leszcz, 2020). The development of specific types of social skills may vary depending on the group's focus. The author's group work with Black Americans has involved a range of social skills development. While conducting a cognitive-behavioral group therapy session, the author has often seen Black group members share feedback regarding ways to deal effectively or communicate with individuals who work on behalf of structures: police, judges, attorneys, case workers, probation officers, teachers, etc. Specific feedback from one Black client to another regarding the adoption of behaviors to successfully complete various forms of mandated treatment (Department of Children Services [DCS], Probation, etc.), while also obtaining their personal goals (freedom from community monitoring, regaining custody of their children) is sometimes provided among Black group members. The feedback on communication and behavior that is shared among Black group members may not be fundamentally different from what is communicated from referral sources (DCS, probation). However, the fact that the feedback comes from a trusted member of the Black community may sometimes have more weight and authenticity than a paid employee.

In group therapy, group members may adopt the same mannerisms and/or behaviors of the group therapist or other group members (Yalom & Leszcz, 2020). In cognitive-behavioral group therapy sessions involving Black group members, the author has seen a Black individual who is new to the group therapy session initially be quieter and more reserved. However, after seeing other Black group members actively participating in the CBT exercises and self-disclosing, the Black individual has at times imitated the proactive participation in cognitive-behavioral group therapy sessions. Yalom's therapeutic factor of imitative behavior is of particular importance when it comes to demonstrating vulnerability. Vulnerability in group therapy could be seen in one Black group member transparently sharing their thoughts and beliefs in the group. The Black group member's demonstrated introspection and vulnerability with sharing their thoughts and beliefs may provide a good model for other Black individuals who are new to the group or reluctant to become vulnerable and share their thoughts and beliefs.

The socially appropriate release of emotion in group therapy is referred to as catharsis and is considered one of Yalom's therapeutic factors (Yalom & Leszcz, 2020). Catharsis is especially important for the Black community, given a tendency for Black men (Taylor et al., 2019) and women (Motro et al., 2022) to be inaccurately and one-dimensionally viewed as angry. Regrettably, in American society, Black men and women are often held to a standard of not showing anger as an emotion. This Procrustean emotional constraint socially precludes Black men and women from expressing the full continuum of human emotion and doing so brings with it fear, social stigma, and/or condemnation. Group therapy, which allows Black men and women to experience and convey the full range of human emotion, without condemnation or fear, can be particularly helpful and healing.

Cohesiveness involves the experience of the group member being connected to other group members and the group clinician (Yalom & Leszcz, 2020). Cohesiveness may manifest itself in a number of different ways within cognitive-behavioral group therapy with Black clients. As was stated previously, microaggressions in group therapy occur at a high rate (Kivlighan III et al., 2021). One of the ways in which cohesiveness may be expressed is when the group members raise an issue with the cognitive-behavioral group therapist regarding how a Black client is treated or perceived to have been treated in a group therapy session. In Black therapy groups with high Cohesiveness, the group members may become protective of members of the group, and this protection spurred by cohesiveness can at times be a check against perceived microaggressions by the group facilitator. Alternatively, cohesiveness may also occur when the Black group members hold another group member accountable for how the group member speaks to the cognitive-behavioral group clinician or disrupts the therapeutic milieu of the group.

7.5 Cognitive-Behavioral Group Therapy and RESPPECTUS Principles

Research has shown that the clinicians who demonstrate more racial/ethnic comfort with racial minority clients have better retention rates for both racial minority and White clients (Owen et al., 2017). Owens and associates conceptualized racial/ethnic comfort as the ease with which clinicians are able to discuss therapeutic and cultural identity issues with racial and ethnic minorities. According to Owens and colleagues, racial/ethnic comfort also included the clinician having and maintaining their positive and authentic engagement when the clinician had cultural and value differences with the racial/ethnic minority client. Cultural adaptation involves comprehending how structural racism impacts Black clients and may catalyze distrust (Lee, 2025). The cognitive-behavioral clinician, having understood the history of anti-Black structural racism (see Chap. 2) and its many experiential and cognitive manifestations (see Chap. 6), would at least in theory be more prepared to demonstrate racial comfort when working with Black Americans. Cognitive-behavioral group therapy, in the context of the RESSPECTUS principles, is discussed here, in an effort to ultimately enhance clinicians' racial comfort and decrease microaggressive behaviors with Black American clients.

7.5.1 Principle 1: Resilience and Strength of Black Americans

For Black American youth (Finkelhor et al., 2013; Rivas-Drake et al., 2014; Sandler et al., 2004), females (Abernethy, 2022; Boyd-Franklin, 1991), and males (Eva et al., 2024; Harris et al., 2020; Hines & Steen, 2020; Prasath et al., 2024), there is a strong history of using the strength-based approaches in group therapy. According to Chen and associates (2008), idiosyncratic and common strengths of a racial group can be emphasized in group therapy, and these unique and shared attributes can be used to empower the group members and address problems. In group therapy sessions, consisting exclusively of Black American clients, the identification and mobilization of strengths for addressing psychosocial problems and stressors can be capitalized. The synergy around the individual and collective identification of Black strengths and resilience may arise from shared stories and histories regarding Black achievements. Black group therapy sessions focused on Black strengths may also create Black pride that serves as a counternarrative to negative rhetoric and images that are promulgated about Black individuals and communities (Bell & Harris, 2017; Vontress, 1971).

7.5.2 Principle 2: Empathy for Black Traumatic Events and Stressors

Human beings are capable of empathy; however, for some individuals, unacknowledged and/or unchallenged structural racism can begin to erode empathic responses to others. Research has shown that the degree to which some White individuals empathize with the pain experienced by others is moderated by race (Forgiarini et al., 2011). The authors of this study found that a decreased response to the pain experienced by African individuals was correlated with the White individual's implicit bias. Empathy for Black traumatic events and stressors could very well be enhanced by having other Black members who participate in the same group therapy session to address shared treatment goals (Marmarosh et al., 2020). The potential for other Black group therapy members to validate and be empathic toward traumatic Black experiences and achievements in group members' lives is valuable and further underscores Yalom's therapeutic factor of cohesiveness (Yalom & Leszcz, 2020). Group therapy with Black Americans should be monitored and considered in terms of how additional members may enhance or diminish the group's empathy. It is possible that a Black group member with substantive internalized anti-Black racism may detract from the group's cohesiveness and shared empathy.

7.5.3 Principle 3: Structural Racism—Influences on Presenting Problems, Rapport, and Therapy

Group therapy with Black individuals can certainly have the potential to generate needed empathy for trauma and distress stemming from structural racism. In group therapy, experiences with structural racism and interpretations of these experiences may be shared. Thus far, regarding the cognitive-behavioral RESPPECTUS principles for Black Americans, microlevel factors and interventions have been discussed; however, a two-tiered approach that also addresses the upstream causes of structural racism is necessary (Bartlett et al., 2022). Beyond providing empathy, some practical and beneficial responses to structural racism occur outside of the therapy setting. As Bartlett and others have stated, advocacy and community involvement are also methods for therapeutically addressing stress, racism, and race-related trauma.

7.5.4 Principle 4: Problem-Solving

Given the presence of Black individuals with their own unique and collective strengths (principle 1: *Resilience and Strength of Black Americans*), the brainstorming component of the problem-solving model (D'Zurilla & Nezu, 1999) may be accentuated. The shared racial identity of the Black group members may provide additional insight into resources, strengths, options, perspectives, and social capital that may be used to resolve psychosocial and racial discrimination problems. Beyond the generation of potential solutions, the group format may also be used to more thoroughly examine the potential pros and cons of each solution, thereby resulting in a more considerate choice of which options to adopt to resolve the problem. Problem-solving exercises that take place in Black psychotherapy groups may also provide some accountability with following up on pursuing options that were identified and selected. When engaging in problem-solving, the group therapy format may allow for support and congratulations when goals are not achieved or obtained, respectively. The open discussion of problems may also support Yalom's therapeutic factor of universality, as other group members may become aware that a problem the individual was struggling with is not necessarily unique to them, but it is also experienced by other Black Americans.

7.5.5 Principle 5: Policy Change

Principle 5, *Policy Change* is closely associated with Bartlett et al. (2022) sentiments regarding a call for structural change and not relying solely on microlevel interventions. Black group therapy members are certainly impacted by policy, as policy is related to their having or not having health insurance, copay amount, socioeconomic factors which impact their daily life, transportation, and other factors which impact their lives and the lives of their loved ones. Depending on the nature of treatment, group therapy members may have case managers, therapists, peer supports, or other individuals who can help the group members access advantageous policies which may positively impact their treatment goals and daily functioning or advocate for using policies on behalf of the Black group therapy members.

7.5.6 Principle 6: Evaluating Thoughts and Beliefs

The roles of cognitive restructuring in group therapy have been articulated in CBT manuals as early as 1984 (Sank & Shaffer). Across the various texts and treatment manuals, different authors have described the use of cognitive restructuring in group therapy. Bieling and associates (2022) have discussed group therapy members participating in the Socratic questioning, and this participation aids in objectively challenging a cognitive distortion and builds Yalom's therapeutic factor of altruism (Yalom & Leszcz, 2020). Sank and Shaffer discussed the use of role-plays in cognitive restructuring, where the group members alter in playing the roles of negative thoughts and more reasonable responses to the negative thoughts. In describing the use of cognitive restructuring in group therapy, Sank and Shaffer state that the goal of cognitive restructuring is not to exchange negative thoughts for positive thoughts, but instead to question the thought, to determine if the thought is reasonably objective. As was discussed previously in Chap. 6, the problem with the term, Reasonably Objective, is that what is reasonable may vary from group to group and culture to culture, hence the social construction of reality (Berger & Luckmann, 1966). Recall that Berger and Luckmann maintained that knowledge depended on the collective agreement of groups, and again, the collective agreement of what is true may differ among groups, cultures, and other factors. If the social construction of reality is not considered, Beck's (1976) warning regarding the cognitive-behavioral clinician imposing their own value becomes more probable. The potential benefit of cognitive restructuring in group therapy with Black group members (exclusively Black or partially Black) is that the challenging of thoughts and beliefs via Socratic questions is no longer funneled solely through the perspective of the client and the cognitive-behavioral clinician. In group therapy with Black group members, there are now other perspectives on what constitutes knowledge or social reality. The presence of other Black group members may provide a shared socially constructed reality that can be used to determine if the evidence for and against a thought is reasonable. In effect, the presence of other Black group members may help make that evaluation of thoughts less prone to cognitive-behavioral clinician imposing their own value system.

7.5.7 *Principle 7: Critical Evaluation of Clinical and Other Relevant Research*

Similar to other aspects of CBT, cognitive-behavioral group therapy with Black Americans is under-researched, as stated in the *Cognitive-Behavioral Group Therapy: Clinical Trials with Black Americans* section of this chapter. Critical evaluations of the cognitive-behavioral group therapy research include the fact that systematic reviews have at times combined all non-White research participants into an amalgamized group, where the distinct and important attributes of each non-White group become somewhat reduced. The systematic reviews have sometimes included multiple groups, and while this describes cognitive-behavioral group commonalities across races and/or cultures, the utility of this research for specific non-White racial groups is at times diminished. In systematic reviews where conclusions may be drawn about non-White groups collectively, it is up to the clinician to pick apart and deconstruct what is most relevant for the Black American the clinician is working with. Within group CBT and other forms of CBT, the racially amalgamized systematic reviews at the very least reduce the amount of clinically relevant CBT knowledge that can be shared about Black individuals.

7.5.8 *Principle 8: Truth and Transparency*

The interdependence of the cognitive-behavioral RESPPECTUS principles was previously discussed in Chap. 4. Principle 7, *Critical Evaluation of Clinical and Other Relevant Research*, is very closely linked to principle 8, Truth and Transparency. Once a cognitive-behavioral clinician understands the status of cognitive-behavioral research for Black Americans, the evidence-based research process involves discussing the clinically relevant research with the client to determine the intervention's fit with the client's treatment objectives and values (Drisko, 2014). The Black American client may have a range of views as it pertains to the acceptability of cognitive-behavioral group therapy. If the response to group therapy involves anxiety, the presence of anxiety regarding the client's participation in the therapeutic group process is not that unusual and may be fueled by anxiety related to being embarrassed or excluded by others or fear of being vulnerable with others (Shay, 2021). Anxiety pertaining to group therapy will range across a continuum. The common anxiety associated with group therapy may potentially be exacerbated when discussing the current number of empirical evaluations of group cognitive-behavioral therapy with Black Americans. However, to some extent, this anxiety may be ameliorated by some of the positive findings that have been published (Ali, 2008; Bowe, 2013; Carter et al., 2003; Ward & Brown, 2015). In the author's own facilitation of cognitive-behavioral group therapy, Black American clients typically had some degree of anxiety regarding participating in group therapy. If Black American clients previously experienced group therapy and had positive experiences in group therapy, the anxiety pertaining to engaging in group therapy was substantially lower. This reduced anxiety was likely attributable to anxious thoughts about group therapy having been disconfirmed via evidence to the contrary as well as through habituation. These are the same mechanisms by which exposure and response prevention therapy work (Norton, 2012). In or near the last sessions of group therapy, the author has consistently seen Black American clients reflect on and articulate the contrast between how anxious they were about group therapy initially and the benefits that they ultimately received from group therapy.

7.5.9 Principle 9: Uniqueness of each Black Individual

The implications of principle 9, regarding cognitive-behavioral group therapy, are as follows: each Black American is unique, there's no guarantee that group therapy will always be beneficial for a Black American, regardless of how many Black individuals may be in the group. In exclusively Black and racially heterogeneous groups, the extent to which Yalom's therapeutic factors are realized is dependent upon the individual personalities of the Black and non-Black group members and actualization of Yalom's therapeutic factors is not guaranteed based on race. Black individuals within groups create the potential for Yalom's therapeutic factors to be realized; however, the presence of other Black group members is not by itself a guarantee that Yalom's therapeutic factors will be experienced. Beyond the Black American clients themselves and their respective group members, the experience of Black individuals in cognitive-behavioral group therapy sessions is also influenced by the cognitive-behavioral group facilitator. Recall that group facilitators with racial/ethnic comfort have better retention rates for racial minority and White clients (Owen et al., 2017). Therefore, as it pertains to cognitive-behavioral group therapy, a number of factors influence outcomes, including but not necessarily limited to the Black client, the group members, and the cognitive-behavioral clinician.

7.5.10 Principle 10: Social Support's Import

Cognitive-behavioral group therapy epitomizes principle 10's emphasis on the importance of social support. Outside of cognitive restructuring and behavioral therapy interventions, Yalom and Leszcz (2020) have best conceptualized the therapeutic factors by which other members of the cognitive-behavioral group will foster growth in the Black American client toward his treatment goals. There is certainly some clinical logic that cognitive-behavioral group therapy may give Black Americans clients hope, create a shared space for connection and inclusion, create new skills, increase social support, and provide a sense of belonging (see Yalom & Leszcz, 2020 discussion of cognitive-behavioral group therapy and therapeutic factors). To some extent, in the author's own research, the beneficial experience of

Yalom's therapeutic factors among Black individuals in group therapy has been empirically supported (Gregory Jr. et al., 2025). In essence, the group therapy format provides Black clients opportunities to experience some of the benefits of social support via being in a therapeutic setting with individuals who share some of the same treatment goals as well as various strengths and resources.

7.6 Cognitive-Behavioral Group Therapy—Integrating RESPPECTUS Principles: Summary

This chapter identified the therapeutic mechanisms by which group therapy may achieve its beneficial effects (Yalom & Leszcz, 2020) and the therapeutic factors' application to Black Americans in group therapy. The cognitive-behavioral RESPPECTUS principles for Black Americans were identified, and their application to cognitive-behavioral group therapy was discussed. The final section and chapter (Chap. 8) discuss CBT and the RESPPECTUS principles in the context of the unique needs of Black men, women, and several Black diasporic groups across the continents.

References

Abernethy, A. D. (2022). Spirituality and struggle as sources of strength and power for African American women: Implications for group therapy leadership. In Y. I. Kane, S. M. Masselink, & A. C. Weiss (Eds.), *Women, intersectionality, and power in group psychotherapy leadership* (pp. 18–32). Routledge/Taylor & Francis Group.

Ali, K. M. (2008). *The effects of two marathon group therapy interventions on the levels of depression and state anxiety in African American women infected with HIV/AIDS* (Doctoral dissertation). Retrieved from PsycINFO (3331071).

Bartlett, A., Faber, S., Williams, M., & Saxberg, K. (2022). Getting to the root of the problem: Supporting clients with lived-experiences of systemic discrimination. *Chronic Stress*, 1–10. https://doi.org/10.1177/24705470221139205

Beck, A. T. (1976). Cognitive therapy and the emotional disorders. *Meridian.*

Bell, G. C., & Harris, T. M. (2017). Exploring representations of black masculinity and emasculation on NBC'S parenthood. *Journal of International and Intercultural Communication, 10*(2), 135–152. https://doi.org/10.1080/17513057.2016.1142598

Berger, P. L., & Luckmann, T. (1966). *The social construction of reality: A treatise in the sociology of knowledge*. Anchor Books.

Bieling, P. J., McCabe, R. E., & Antony, M. M. (2022). *Cognitive-behavioral therapy in groups* (2nd ed.). Guilford Press.

Bowe, W. (2013). *Refinement and pilot testing of a culturally enhanced treatment for depressed African Americans. [Doctoral thesis]*. University of Wisconsin-Milwaukee. https://dc.uwm.edu/etd/229

Boyd-Franklin, N. (1991). Recurrent themes in the treatment of African-American women in group psychotherapy. *Women & Therapy, 11*(2), 25–40. https://doi.org/10.1300/J015V11N02_04

Burns, D. D. (1989). *The feeling good handbook*. Penguin Books.

Carter, M. M., Sbrocco, T., Gore, K. L., Marin, N. W., & Lewis, E. L. (2003). Cognitive-behavioral group therapy versus a wait-list control in treatment of African American women with panic disorder. *Cognitive Therapy and Research, 27*(5), 505–518. https://doi.org/10.1023/A:1026350903639

Chen, E. C., Kakkad, D., & Balzano, J. (2008). Multicultural competence and evidence-based practice in group therapy. *Journal of Clinical Psychology, 64*(11), 1261–1278. https://doi.org/10.1002/jclp.20533

D'Zurilla, J. J., & Nezu, A. M. (1999). *Problem-solving therapy: A social competence approach to clinical intervention* (2nd ed.). Springer Publications Company.

Drisko, J. (2014). Research evidence and social work practice: The place of evidence-based practice. *Clinical Social Work Journal, 42*, 123–133. https://doi.org/10.1007/s10615-013-0459-9

Eva, M. G., Cook, M. I., Sandifer, K. R., & Osagie-Ekhovbiye, F. (2024). Group counseling for black male students: A strengths-based approach. *Professional School Counseling, 28*(1). https://doi.org/10.1177/2156759X241234899

Finkelhor, D., Turner, H. A., Shattuck, A., & Hamby, S. L. (2013). Violence, crime, and abuse exposure in a national sample of children and youth: An update. *JAMA Pediatrics, 167*(7), 614–621. https://doi.org/10.1001/jamapediatrics.2013.42

Forgiarini, M., Gallucci, M., & Maravita, A. (2011). Racism and the empathy for pain on our skin. *Frontiers in Psychology, 2*, 108. https://doi.org/10.3389/fpsyg.2011.00108

Gregory, V. L., Jr., Zapolski, T., Marriott, B. R., Lipsey, A., Hicks, A. I., & Lee, C. (2025). *Exploring the lived experience of Black Americans and substance use treatment: Structural, community, and individual factors*. [Manuscript submitted]. School of Social Work, Indiana University.

Harris, P. C., Mayes, R. D., Freeman, C., Eberly, B., Tatby, N., & Wiener, S. (2020). Men passionately pursuing purpose (MP3): A group counseling intervention for black male student athletes. *Journal for Specialists in Group Work, 45*(2), 146–164. https://doi.org/10.1080/01933922.2019.1679931

Hines, E. M., & Steen, S. (2020). Group work with black/African American males. *Journal for Specialists in Group Work, 45*(2), 97–98. https://doi.org/10.1080/01933922.2020.1745496

Joe, J. R., Shillingford-Butler, M. A., & Oh, S. (2019). The experiences of African American mothers raising sons in the context of #BlackLivesMatter. *The Professional Counselor, 9*(1), 67–79. https://doi.org/10.15241/jrj.9.1.67

Kivlighan, D. M., III, Swancy, A. G., Smith, E., & Brennaman, C. (2021). Examining racial microaggressions in group therapy and the buffering role of members' perceptions of their group's multicultural orientation. *Journal of Counseling Psychology, 68*(5), 621–628. https://doi.org/10.1037/cou0000531

Kohn, L. P., Oden, T., Munoz, R. F., Robinson, A., & Leavitt, D. (2002). Adapted cognitive behavioral group therapy for depressed low-income African American women. *Community Mental Health Journal, 38*, 497–504. https://doi.org/10.1023/a:1020884202677

Kunorubwe, T. (2023). Cultural adaptations of group CBT for depressed clients from diverse backgrounds: A systematic review. *The Cognitive Behaviour Therapist, 16*, e35. https://doi.org/10.1017/S1754470X23000302

Lee, C. (2025). *Motivational interviewing across cultures: Optimizing practice*. Guilford Press.

Lui, P. P., & Quezada, L. (2019). Associations between microaggression and adjustment outcomes: A meta-analytic and narrative review. *Psychological Bulletin, 145*(1), 45–78. https://doi.org/10.1037/bul0000172

Marmarosh, C. L., Forsyth, D. R., Strauss, B., & Burlingame, G. M. (2020). The psychology of the COVID-19 pandemic: A group-level perspective. *Group Dynamics: Theory, Research, and Practice, 24*(3), 122–138. https://doi.org/10.1037/gdn0000142

Miles, J. R., Anders, C., Kivlighan, D. M., III, & Belcher Platt, A. A. (2021). Cultural ruptures: Addressing microaggressions in group therapy. *Group Dynamics: Theory, Research, and Practice, 25*(1), 74–88. https://doi.org/10.1037/gdn0000149

Motro, D., Evans, J. B., Ellis, A. P. J., & Benson, L. I. I. I. (2022). Race and reactions to women's expressions of anger at work: Examining the effects of the "angry black woman" stereotype. *Journal of Applied Psychology, 107*(1), 142–152. https://doi.org/10.1037/apl0000884

Nichols, M. P., & Davis, S. D. (2017). *Family therapy: Concepts and methods* (11th ed.). Pearson.

Norton, P. J. (2012). *Group cognitive-behavioral therapy of anxiety: A transdiagnostic treatment manual*. Guilford Press.

Owen, J., Drinane, J., Tao, K. W., Adelson, J. L., Hook, J. N., Davis, D., & Fookune, N. (2017). Racial/ethnic disparities in client unilateral termination: The role of therapists' cultural comfort. *Psychotherapy Research, 27*(1), 102–111. https://doi.org/10.1080/10503307.2015.1078517

Prasath, P. R., Steen, S., & McVay, K. (2024). A creative strengths-based group counseling intervention for African American boys. *Journal of Creativity in Mental Health, 19*(2), 232–243. https://doi.org/10.1080/15401383.2023.2166184

Pierce, C. M., Carew, J. V., Pierce-Gonzalez, D., & Wills, D. (1977). An experiment in racism: Tv commercials. *Education & Urban Society, 10*(1), 61–87. https://doi.org/10.1177/001312457701000105

Rivas-Drake, D., Seaton, E. K., Markstrom, C., Quintana, S., Syed, M., Lee, R. M., & Yip, T. (2014). Ethnic and racial identity in adolescence: Implications for psychosocial, academic, and health outcomes. *Child Development, 85*, 40–57. https://doi.org/10.1111/cdev.12200

Sandler, I. N., Ayers, T. S., Suter, J. C., Schultz, A., & Twohey-Jacobs, J. (2004). Adversities, strengths, and public policy. In K. I. Maton, C. J. Schellenbach, B. J. Leadbeater, & A. L. Solarz (Eds.), *Investing in children, youth, families, and communities: Strengths-based research and policy* (pp. 31–49). American Psychological Association.

Sank, L. I., & Shaffer, C. S. (1984). *A therapist's manual for cognitive behavior therapy in groups*. Plenum Press.

Shay, J. J. (2021). Terrified of group therapy: Investigating obstacles to entering or leading groups. *American Journal of Psychotherapy, 74*(2), 71–75. https://doi.org/10.1176/appi.psychotherapy.20200033

Stack, C. (1983). *All our kin: Strategies for survival in a Black community*. Basic Books.

Taylor, E., Guy-Walls, P., Wilkerson, P., & Addae, R. (2019). The historical perspectives of stereotypes on African-American males. Journal of human. *Rights and Social Work, 4*, 213–225. https://doi.org/10.1007/s41134-019-00096-y

Ward, E. C., & Brown, R. L. (2015). A culturally adapted depression intervention for African American adults experiencing depression: Oh, happy day. *American Journal of Orthopsychiatry, 85*, 11–22. https://doi.org/10.1037/ort0000027

Webb Hooper, M., Antoni, M. H., Okuyemi, K., Dietz, N. A., & Resnicow, K. (2017). Randomized controlled trial of group-based culturally specific cognitive behavioral therapy among African American smokers. *Nicotine & Tobacco Research, 19*(3), 333–341. https://doi.org/10.1093/ntr/ntw181

Vontress, C. E. (1971). Racial differences: Impediments to rapport. *Journal of Counseling Psychology, 18*(1), 7–13. https://doi.org/10.1037/h0030758

Yalom, I. D., & Leszcz, M. (2020). *The theory and practice of group psychotherapy* (6th ed.). Basic Books/Hachette Book Group.

Part III
RESPPECTUS Principles: Applications to Black Demographic Groups

Chapter 8
Cognitive-Behavioral Therapy: Black Men, Women, and Black Diasporic Groups

8.1 Cognitive-Behavioral Therapy (CBT) with Black American Men: RESPPECTUS Principles

8.1.1 Strength and Resilience of Black American Men

Despite negative images and stereotypes, in the United States Black men have a broad array of strengths and resilience that may be mobilized to address mental illness and other psychosocial problems (principle 1: *Resilience and Strength of Black Americans*). Research with Black men has documented their strength and resilience across a number of circumstances and conditions. In a midwestern qualitative study examining Black men's coping following the traumatic murder of George Floyd, Black men were shown to have used: reframing or cognitive restructuring, spiritual and religious resources, different forms of social support, social media technology for social change and mental well-being (Gregory Jr. & Tucker Edmonds, 2023). The same study showed Black men has having an enduring positive self-image that was robust to negative perceptions and structural inequity, as well as using self-reflection to facilitate constructive change. A qualitative study by Teti et al. (2012) examined the resilience of Black men in Philadelphia and found similar key aspects of resilience that included: religious and spiritual support, intrapersonal and interpersonal support, personal growth and development, self-reflection and change. Chung et al.'s (2014) qualitative study explored factors that support resiliency in Black men in Los Angeles, also showing themes of faith and spirituality, as well as familial and other social support.

Quantitative research (Thomas Tobin et al., 2022,) which has categorized and compared Black male strengths or resources with regard to physiological well-being has found two categories of psychosocial resources or strengths that contribute to physiological resilience. These two categories of strengths or resources share some similarities with the strengths and resilience factors seen in qualitative

V. L. Gregory, Jr., *Cognitive-Behavioral Therapy with Black Americans*,
https://doi.org/10.1007/978-3-032-01666-9_8

research. The first class consisted of Black men who have high resources. These resources in the first category included high levels of: belief that God had control over their lives, perceived familial support, perceived support from friends, self-efficacy, and high levels of racial identity. The second category included Black men with minimal resources but high self-efficacy. In this second category, Black men were low on: religious coping, belief that God had control over their lives, racial identity, and social support. The authors of the study concluded that the two categories of Black male strengths or resources had symbiotic relationships with one another that collectively accounted for physiological resilience among Black American men. In addition to strengths and resilience, the same studies have also shown Black male stressors associated with racism, financial problems, legal issues, or other structural factors (Chung et al., 2014; Gregory Jr. & Tucker Edmonds, 2023; Teti et al., 2012).

What does the extant qualitative and quantitative research tell us about Black men, their strengths and resilience, and the implications for CBT principles? The strengths and resilience factors identified in the extant research show thematic overlap with the cognitive-behavioral RESPPECTUS principles for Black Americans. The Black male strength-based behavioral science literature supports the RESPPECTUS principles as it relates to spiritual strengths (principle 1: *Resilience and Strength of Black Americans*), the detrimental impact of structural racism (principle 3: *Structural Racism—Influences on Presenting Problems, Rapport, and Therapy*), self-efficacy (principle 4: *Problem-Solving*), and social support (principle 10: *Social Support's Import*).

In this chapter, a number of Black American male strengths have been identified through research. The identified strengths of Black American men in this chapter are not exhaustive and vary among Black men. All Black men have strengths and the capacity for resilience. In accordance with principle 9 (*Uniqueness of Each Black Individual*) strengths and the ability of each Black man to mobilize those strengths vary from person to person. It is the function of the cognitive-behavioral therapist to facilitate the exploration, identification, and utilization of Black male strengths to inform cognitive-behavioral conceptualizations and interventions.

8.1.2 Structurally Determined Black Male Health Disparities and Cognitive-Behavioral Therapy

Principle 3 (*Structural Racism—Influences on Presenting Problems, Rapport, and Therapy*), calls for the CBT clinician to take into account the impact of structural racism on the Black male client's presenting issue, therapeutic rapport, and CBT interventions. In Chap. 2, the structural context of CBT with Black American men and women was described wholistically. This section addresses the structural influence on the lives of Black American men and its specific implications for health disparities and CBT. The Centers for Disease Control and Prevention (CDC, 2024) defines health disparities as differences in the total number of cases with a disease, the number of new cases with a disease, and mortality from disease based on race, gender, and other demographic traits. Black men have been disproportionately represented in risk factors for chronic illnesses such as heart disease and various psychiatric conditions, and have been considered the most at-risk group for health disparities in the United States (Okoro et al., 2020). An exhaustive list of all the health disparities among Black men is beyond the scope of this text. However, it is important to note, the wide array of Black male health disparities in the US suggests a broader structural foundation that undergirds or even causes and maintains these health disparities. The structural foundation of health disparities among Black men in America is those US laws, policies, institutions, and practices that were discussed in Chap. 2 of the present text.

How does structural racism impact CBT with Black American men? A structural equation model has shown that structural racism (Tripartite Police Fear) was related to perceived cultural barriers to mental health treatment for Black American men (Gregory et al., in press). The structural equation model used the Tripartite Police Fear and the Beliefs about American and Its Justice System subscales of the Cultural Trauma Scale (Gregory Jr. & Tucker Edmonds, 2024b), available in Appendix D. The Cultural Barriers subscale came from the Barriers to Seeking Mental Health Counseling scale (Shea et al., 2019). In this model, as Black men's Tripartite Police Fear increased their perceptions of cultural barriers to accessing professional mental health treatment also increased (Gregory et al., in press). While this empirical relationship does not infer causation, the theory that cultural trauma (deriving from structural racism) predicts or even causes health disparities has been logically reasoned and described (Subica & Link, 2022). As scales that measure components of structural racism (see Table 4.1 in Chap. 4) become more prominent, statistical modeling of these latent variables and their relationships to Black male mental health treatment is likely to increase. Extant research explains the structural mechanisms by which Black men and women may have concerns about mental health treatment (Shim, 2021). However, in accordance with principle 9 (*Uniqueness of Each Black Individual*), these concerns will vary depending on the specific Black man the CBT clinician is working with. The nature and unique history of CBT do not mitigate these concerns. In fact, CBT's lack of external validity, as it pertains to non-White individuals (Huey Jr et al., 2023), may exacerbate some of these concerns.

8.1.3 Empathy for Black Male Traumatic Events and Stressors in CBT

The first, CBT-relevant concern of structural racism is one of engagement as Black men may not participate in professional mental health treatment due to distrust of systems (Gregory Jr. & Clary, 2022). Engagement in psychotherapy can be defined in multiple ways: attendance, participation, homework completion, and the clinician's therapeutic rapport with the client (Holdsworth et al., 2014). As it pertains to attendance, approximately one-half to three-fourths of Black men who have experienced trauma may not have received necessary mental health treatment (Motley & Banks, 2018). In one study, Black women and men were reluctant to participate in mental health treatment; however, men were significantly less willing to obtain mental health treatment (Ward et al., 2013). In another study, 80% of the interviews involved Black men discussing their unwillingness to process racial injustice issues with professional helpers (Gregory Jr. & Tucker Edmonds, 2023). These men cited their preference to speak to a pastor and lack of financial resources as influential factors. Self-stigma (Shannon, 2023) has been shown to be an indicator of decreased attendance in mental health treatment. Other research has shown that as psychological hardiness increases, help-seeking among Black men also increases (Cadaret & Speight, 2018).

The available research examining Black men's willingness to participate in psychotherapy is important given its implications for treatment targets, interventions, and the therapeutic relationship in CBT. The behavioral science literature, examining barriers to engagement, is useful because it provides some context for what Black American men may be experiencing and thinking when they do arrive for their first CBT session. Decades ago, Vontress (1971) stated that black men were the most marginalized in the US. Based on more recent social, economic, medical, and legal disparities in the United States, Black men are still erroneously considered the least valuable members of American society. Historically, within the United States, Black men have been viewed as inherently unsuccessful, oversexed, criminal, and aggressive (Bell & Harris, 2017). This overarching and inaccurate view of Black men as negative lays the social foundation for Black men to be disregarded, discounted, and disrespected in psychotherapy and other healthcare and social venues of American society. The author has experience with providing CBT to Black men, conducting research with Black men, and speaking to Black men in formal and informal settings regarding the intersection of social injustice and mental illness. The recurrent theme across these clinical, empirical, and public/personal settings is for Black men to be treated with respect in mental health treatment and healthcare services overall.

In CBT, a primary need is for Black men to be authentically viewed and treated with dignity and respect. Qualitative research has underscored the importance of respect for Black clients, from mental health providers (Earl et al., 2011). Earl and colleagues study found that Black clients believed that respect was in part demonstrated via the providers not judging Black clients. In the same study, a Black male client, referring to his provider, discussed how he refused to work with the provider due to the providers lack of reciprocated respect for the Black male client. Principle 2 (*Empathy for Black Traumatic Events and Stressors*) embodies the need for respect to be communicated in a genuine and absolute manner when working with Black men. In consideration of the essential therapeutic rapport component of CBT with Black men and women, the acronym for the CBT principles was aptly given the name RESPPECTUS, pronounced "Respect Us."

Where does respect for Black men begin in CBT? Respect for Black men in CBT certainly includes the four clinician factors identified by Rogers (1957): Being invested in the relationship, comprehending the client's experience, having unconditional positive regard for the client, and communicating expressions of the client's experience. Providing the Black male client with an opportunity to discuss past microaggressive experiences in therapy (Hankerson et al., 2015) is also another way to demonstrate respect and build therapeutic rapport. Cognitive-behavioral therapy is didactic and collaborative (Leahy, 1996). In discussing the rationale for CBT with Black men, the CBT clinician should discuss some of the distinctive features of CBT, the session structure, expectations of CBT, and the RESPPECTUS principles that are being used. This discussion would serve as education, so the Black male client has more knowledge regarding what is expected in CBT. The Black male client can also ask substantive questions or provide feedback regarding the clinician's adherence to or departure from CBT and the RESPPECTUS principles. Beck (2021) has recommended the overt elicitation of client feedback throughout CBT sessions. This too demonstrates respect and the collaborative nature of CBT by routinely seeking feedback from the Black male client regarding his perception of the CBT process. As stated before, for the CBT clinician to develop and maintain sufficient therapeutic rapport with and respect for the Black male client, the CBT clinician must first have honest introspection and self-awareness of the clinician's own perceptions of Black men. The CBT clinician should be aware of where those perceptions come from and how the CBT clinician's perceptions of Black people and culture are consistent with and contrary to the actual lived experience of the Black American man with whom the clinician is working with.

The distrust of systems, created by structural racism should also be included in the CBT clinician's CBT conceptualization of and work with the Black male client. There are varying degrees of perceived structural racism that may be present, from none up to a lot! Several ways of quantifying perceptions of structural racism are through the Cultural Trauma Scale's America and Its Justice System: Cognitive-Emotional Responses (see Appendix C, Gregory Jr. & Tucker Edmonds, 2024a), Beliefs about American and Its Justice System (see Appendix D, Gregory Jr. & Tucker Edmonds, 2024b), and Tripartite Police Fear (Gregory Jr. & Tucker Edmonds, 2024a, 2024b) subscales. It has been previously stated that distrust created by structural racism may undermine Black men's and women's participation in systems that may be non-adversarial and truly beneficial for them (Gregory Jr. & Clary, 2022).

For Black men with greater police fear, matters of respect, and therapeutic rapport may become even more important given the Black male client's own potential beliefs about therapy and the psychotherapy enterprise (Gregory et al., in press). For example, when working with Black men who were court-ordered for substance use treatment, the author was routinely told, "you're only here for the money!" While the author's intentions were to aid and advocate for the Black male client in achieving his goals, the client was participating in a court system where the client believed the primary focus was monetary and punitive rather than rehabilitative. As outlined in Chap. 2, *The Structural Context of Cognitive-Behavioral Therapy with Black Americans*, the mass incarceration of subsequent denial of rights for Black men has been legitimately viewed as an indirect means of keeping Black citizens from making economic, social, and intrapersonal progress (Alexander, 2010). So, while some of the Black male clients' perceptions of the author where not commensurate with the author's actual intentions, the reasoning behind their beliefs was understandable and aligned with history and contemporary dominant structural forces. It is incumbent upon the CBT clinician to center the Black male client's experience with systems and structures and to build a therapeutic rapport that is robust to initial client distrust, which may dissipate over time. Clinical work with the Black male client, using CBT and the RESPPECTUS principles, may provide an experience with the Black male client that may disconfirm his negative beliefs about the therapeutic process and/or the therapist.

8.1.4 Cognitive Restructuring with Black American Men

System 1 and 2 thinking provides a substantive framework for considering the use of cognitive restructuring with Black men and women. A bestselling book by Daniel Kahneman (2011), *Thinking, Fast and Slow*, distinguishes two types of thinking: Systems 1 and 2. To reiterate, the former is quick, efficient, automatic thinking that is prone to errors or cognitive biases when making decisions. To the contrary, System 2 is slow, deliberate, and catches thinking errors that are present in System 1. As previously stated, there are negative and detrimental stereotypes that exist regarding Black men in American culture (Taylor et al., 2019). It is conceivable that clinical decisions in CBT could be made that are not grounded in truth or the Black male client's best interest when System 1 thinking is being used by the cognitive-behavioral clinician. The use of the 10 RESPPECTUS cognitive-behavioral principles is provided to further facilitate System 2 thinking of CBT clinicians as it pertains to treatment with Black American men and women. Erroneous and dominant stereotypes of Black men as emotionally one-dimensional (anger-driven) or lacking introspection to engage in cognitive restructuring are not supported by empirical evidence (Gregory Jr. & Tucker Edmonds, 2023). Principle 6 (*Evaluating Thoughts and Beliefs*) applies to Black men because the cognitive model, which suggest that distorted thinking results in distorted emotions and behavior is certainly applicable (Beck, 2021). When using cognitive restructuring with Black men it is essential to:

- Develop and sustain a therapeutic rapport that facilitates vulnerable discussions of thoughts and beliefs that may be contrary to traditionally held Black male masculinity,
- Conduct a thorough biopsychosocial assessment that informs the cognitive-behavioral case formulation,
- Co-create a well-developed cognitive-behavioral case formulation; elicit and incorporate the Black male client's feedback on the case formulation,
- Provide education on the cognitive model (see Chap. 6),
- Provide a substantive rationale for cognitive interventions that are based on the cognitive model.

8.1.5 Barriers to Accessing Social Support for Black American Men

Principle 10 (*Social Support's Import*) calls for the use of the Black client's social support network and social resources to further advance the client's mental health and treatment goals. Longstanding commonly held notions of Black manhood/masculinity may potentially impede the Black male client's access to some social supports that may otherwise be available. For example, the Black male client may have parents, siblings, spouse, significant other, friends, fraternal brothers, mentors, or other social supports that may be willing and able to provide various forms of assistance the Black male client may benefit from. However, thoughts that negatively distort the true nature of Black male masculinity or manhood may prevent the Black man from using these potentially helpful social supports. These negative thoughts about Black manhood or masculinity may in part derive from popular media (Bell & Harris, 2017), familial beliefs that are passed down through generations, socially accepted and unchallenged understandings of what Black masculinity is or should be within one Black man's specific generation, and other sources.

The thought or belief that accessing social support or seeking help is not consistent with Black masculinity or manhood could very well be the focus of a cognitive intervention. Using Ellis's (1994) ABCD (Activating Event, Beliefs, Consequences, Disputation) model, in cognitive restructuring, each of the three components (negative definitions of Black masculinity based on popular media, family, and peers) would be considered activating events (A). The negative beliefs that Black men have about their own masculinity would be the cognitive content (B) that the cognitive interventions (D) would focus on. The behavioral consequences of the negative, internalized beliefs regarding Black masculinity would be the Black man refusing to obtain or fully accessing potentially helpful social supports (C). The emotional consequence of the Black man's negative beliefs regarding manhood would potentially be guilt or shame (C) associated with reasonable requests for help or assistance. Once the notion that Black masculinity or manhood is incompatible with seeking help has been replaced, the CBT clinician can aid the Black male client in developing the skills to request help. These skills could include assertiveness training, other communication skills, role-playing to practice the skills and receive feedback, and identifying resources within the community that may provide the necessary help the Black male client needs.

8.1.6 Social Policy and Black American Men: Implications for CBT

Principle 5 (*Policy Change*) involves the CBT clinician using their expertise to advance policy-oriented issues that beneficially influence Black Americans. Many of the issues that Black men may present in CBT such as trauma and substance use can be linked to policies that create and sustain mental health disparities among Black males in America. Laws and policies that collectively contribute to the mass incarceration and legal disenfranchisement (Alexander, 2010) of Black men have an enduring impact on a broad array of mental health disparities which impact Black American men. The CBT clinician's understanding of laws and social policies which disenfranchise Black men can aid in understanding the structural realities which may create and sustain many of the micro-level issues that Black men may want or need to address in their CBT sessions. This understanding of laws and policies which impact Black American men could also be beneficial in creating empathy (principle 2: *Empathy for Black Traumatic Events and Stressors*) regarding Black male distrust of systems, such as the mental healthcare system. The understanding of laws and social policy also provides CBT clinicians with important contextual insight, which may enable greater understanding of Black male clients' socially constructed realities and experiences, which may influence their core beliefs and thoughts.

Beyond empathy and cognition, understanding the role of laws and policy in impacting the lives of Black American men receiving CBT can aid in case and class advocacy. Cognitive-behavioral therapists come from different helping professions with each providing its unique contribution to the conceptualization of problems which Black men face in America. Each of the helping professions include CBT clinicians who belong to different professional organizations, communities, and social organizations where advocacy can be used to advance understanding and policy regarding Black men and the clinically oriented problems they address in CBT sessions. These clinical issues include various forms of trauma and racism, mental health and substance use issues, forensic issues, and other psychosocial difficulties that are treated with CBT. Some CBT clinicians are also skilled clinical researchers, and these empirical skills can also be used to inform CBT practice with Black American men. Research investigating clinically relevant questions pertaining to Black men can also be used for advocacy and policy change.

8.2 Cognitive-Behavioral Therapy with Black American Women: RESPPECTUS Principles

8.2.1 Resilience and Strength of Black American Women

In a scoping review addressing the resilience of Black American women, resilience was defined as adaptability to various stressors via the use of interpersonal resources/relationships, coping skills, exercise, community, financial, self-care, and spiritual resources (Woods-Giscombe et al., 2023). This definition of resilience, pertaining to Black American women, is aligned with the cognitive-behavioral RESPPECTUS principles for Black Americans. The congruence between the resilience of Black American women and the cognitive-behavioral RESPPECTUS principles is particularly evident as it relates to the principles' focus on cognitive restructuring (principle 6: Evaluating Thoughts and Beliefs), social/communal (principle 10: *Social Support's Import*), and spiritual (principle 1: *Resilience and Strength of Black Americans*), aspects of Black Americans and their rather unique historical and social juxtaposition in the US.

Cognitive-behavioral therapy has been considered by some to potentially be less effective with Black American women because of the focus on symptoms while neglecting the cultural, social, and historical context that catalyze the symptoms (Abrams et al., 2019). Abrams and associates maintain that CBT and other therapeutic approaches may treat strength as a pathology without acknowledging the function it serves in the lives of Black women. Black women's strengths have been considered in their practical ability to provide a buffer against racialized stressors via Black women acknowledging the strength of each other in their communications to one another (Davis, 2018). The Strong Black Woman concept, has received considerable empirical and literary attention in behavioral and social science. The concept has been indicative of detrimental coping and diminished mental health (West et al., 2016).

As it pertains to principle 1 (*Resilience and Strength of Black Americans*), the RESPPECTUS principles do not endorse or suggest the use of the Strong Black Woman (Beauboeuf-Lafontant, 2008) or Superwoman Schema (Leath et al., 2023) during the provision of CBT with Black American women. Principle 1, as it pertains to Black American women, does acknowledge that Black women, similar to every other racial and gender demographic, do possess strengths and resilience, and these attributes can be beneficially utilized in the course of CBT. In Chap. 4, the interdependence of the 10 cognitive-behavioral principles for Black Americans was discussed. This interdependent relationship of the RESPPECTUS principles is especially demonstrated in the identification and use of Black women's strength and resilience in CBT. With Black American women, strengths and resilience, which is mobilized in Principle 1, should also be balanced by the social context (principle 3: *Structural Racism—Influences on Presenting Problems, Rapport, and Therapy*) and unique needs (principle 9: *Uniqueness of Each Black Individual*) of the Black American women as was suggested by Abrams and associates (2019). The need to validate and empathize with Black American women (principle 2: *Empathy for Black Traumatic Events and Stressors*) who do have considerable strengths and resilience yet are socialized to inhibit expressions of vulnerability or to project strength which may be self-destructive (Leath et al., 2023) is crucial in CBT and may help mitigate some of the CBT criticisms laid out by Abrams and colleagues. Principle 10 (*Social Support's Import*) can also be utilized with Black American women to underscore the importance of reciprocal-symbiotic relationships. In reciprocal-symbiotic relationships, both members of any interpersonal dyad give and receive support and both receive mutual benefit.

8.2.2 Structural Racism and its Impact on Black American Women in CBT

Principle 3: *Structural Racism—Influences on Presenting Problems, Rapport, and Therapy*, has important nuances when applying it to Black American women. Structural racism is associated with numerous health disparities that disproportionately affect morbidity and treatment engagement for Black American women. Examples include severe adverse maternal outcomes (Guglielminotti et al., 2024), triple negative breast cancer (Eldridge & Berrigan, 2022), obesity and higher diastolic blood pressure (Basile Ibrahim et al., 2021), coronary heart disease (Sheehy et al., 2024), and participation in human immunodeficiency viruses (HIV) health services (Randolph et al., 2020) among others. Structural racism not only manifests itself in diverse healthcare disparities, but also in police violence against Black women. Women are often only considered peripherally in public discussions regarding anti-Black police violence (Joseph, 2022; Willingham, 2018). However, recent highly publicized police killings of Black American women such as Atatiana Jefferson (Smith, 2021), Breonna Taylor (Cecil, 2024), and Sonya Massey (Sangamon County, Illinois, 2024) have provided more attention and structural scrutiny. Research has substantiated the fact that structural racism and subsidiary anti-Black police violence have a substantial and deleterious impact on Black women in America. These studies have documented the trauma Black women experience from seeing police violence against the Black American community on social media (Williams, 2021), fear that Black women have for their sons being victims of police violence (Mehra et al., 2022), fear regarding navigating the complexity of explaining anti-Black racism to their children (Coates et al., 2024), fear and distrust of police regarding the Black woman's reporting intimate partner violence (Sharpless et al., 2024), and Black women being killed by police at higher numbers relative to their White female counterparts (Edwards et al., 2019). Similar to health disparities among Black men, the collection of enduring, non-isolated health disparities among Black women in America suggests a systemic or structural cause. Empirical research has also found an association between Black women being exposed to police violence and increased risk of hypertension (Talbert, 2023), suggesting a pernicious compounding effect between the two manifestations of structural racism (healthcare and anti-Black police violence).

It is theoretically plausible that, similar to Black American men (Gregory et al., in press), structural racism may create perceived cultural barriers to mental health treatment and negatively influence Black women's engagement and retention in mental health treatment. The Center for Behavioral Health Statistics and Quality (2021) examined the rates at which utilization of any mental health treatment and treatment for severe mental illness differed by race and gender, between the years of 2015–2019. Their examination found that Black women have consistently obtained mental health services (treatment for any mental illness and treatment for severe mental illness) more often the Black men. Yet the use of mental health services by Black American women was still less than that of their White male and female counterparts. For Black women of reproductive age, decreased participation in mental health treatment can in part be explained by age and structurally influenced factors such as lack of insurance and decreased education (Ash et al., 2024). This same study also found that for Black women who had obtained mental health treatment, over half had mental health needs which were not fully addressed.

What are the CBT implications of anti-Black structural racism for Black women? Due to structural factors such as laws, policies, and institutions, some Black women may come to CBT with complex needs that extend beyond the presenting diagnostic issue. Due to structural racism, distrust for the cognitive-behavioral clinician and the healthcare system may exist, and this distrust may be a barrier to developing a therapeutic rapport that is necessary for the CBT process. Identifying and sharing thoughts and beliefs require vulnerability. Black women, like their male counterparts, may have some substantive distrust regarding sharing cognitive content that derives from introspection and self-analysis. Black women in CBT may have particular fear about divulging information regarding their substance use or experiences with intimate partner violence due to a perceived fear that the Black women may be reported to a child protective service agency or even lose their children (Smith & Roane, 2023). The Black women's fears of being reported to child protective services are warranted as empirical research shows that Black children, relative to White children, are disparately overrepresented in the substantiation of maltreatment and placement in foster care (Briggs et al., 2022). Briggs and colleagues concluded that racism was a key factor in the child protective services disparities. Boyd (2022) has also argued that structural racism has a pivotal role in disproportionate, racially biased reporting in child welfare. Cognitive-behavioral therapist will need to be receptive to the unique experiences and perspectives of Black women, as well as knowledgeable about the research base regarding structural racism and structural racism's detrimental impact on Black clients. Cognitive-behavioral clinicians, when working with Black women, must consider the objective reality that is evidenced in social science as well as the socially constructed realities (Berger & Luckmann, 1966) that are evidenced in the Black client's experiences and communication.

8.2.3 Empathy with Black Women in CBT: Self-Disclosure

A Black woman's distrust in psychotherapy could derive from the institution of psychotherapy, the therapeutic processes, the specific provider of CBT, and structural racism which may pervade the therapeutic alliance. The potential fears and distrust of Black women receiving CBT are supported by the empirical literature, as cited above, and/or the Black woman's own personal lived experience. This fear and distrust is best addressed by the cognitive-behavioral clinician's empathic response (principle 2) and his truth and transparency (principal 8). Principle 2 (*Empathy for Black Traumatic Events and Stressors*) calls for the CBT clinician's overt expressions of empathy to Black women's experiences and perceptions of these experiences.

Beyond traditional therapeutic techniques for conveying empathy (Egan & Reese, 2019) and engaging clients in the early phases of the therapeutic process (Miller & Rollnick, 2023), self-disclosure (Constantine & Kwan, 2003) has been used as a potential way to improve empathy and engagement with both Black female and male clients. Constantine and Kwan define therapist self-disclosure as things a behavioral health provider may say or do that provide private information about the therapist to their client. A non-Black cognitive-behavioral clinician may self-disclose a number of things in an effort to build a therapeutic rapport with or convey empathy to a Black female client. For example, a non-Black provider of CBT may:

- State that their spouse is Black.
- Say that their children or grandchildren are Black or biracial.
- State that they grew up poor in a predominantly Black neighborhood where they were one of the few Whites with many Black friends.
- Discuss his humanitarian mission trips to impoverished African nations.
- Have pictures in his office at a social event with Black friends.

The above examples are all instances of self-disclosure that may be used proactively or retroactively to build rapport or to salvage therapeutic rapport, respectively. Constatine and Kwan have discussed some of the potential clinical advantages of provider self-disclosure for therapeutic rapport. As it pertains to Principle 8, *Truth and Transparency*, the clinician may self-disclose their relative lack of experience in working with Black women and this could amplify the Black woman's fear, distrust, or cynicism regarding participating in CBT with that clinician. Alternatively, that specific self-disclosure may foster an honest discussion of race and its potential implications for CBT moving forward. Such an instance may further break the barrier of discussing racially sensitive issues in CBT. However, there are some clinical risks in the self-disclosure of non-Black CBT clinicians to Black female and male clients. Some Black female and male clients may potentially take offense to different forms of the CBT clinician's self-disclosure. The Black client may believe that the racial content of the CBT clinician's self-disclosure may be associating Black culture and identity with stereotypical depictions of Black Americans as poor or needy or inferior in some way. If the Black client believes that the CBT clinician's self-disclosure is offensive or stereotypical, this perception will likely stifle the therapeutic rapport necessary for CBT and would be contrary to principle 9 (*Uniqueness of Each Black Individual*), hence the clinical risk of clinician self-disclosure in CBT. How the CBT clinician's self-disclosures pertaining to race are perceived and whether it is viewed as helpful or harmful is ultimately determined by the Black client.

It is important to note that simply being a Black (racially concordant) CBT clinician does not always mean that the Black female or Black male client will have trust or a good therapeutic rapport. For example, a Black male CBT clinician may be working with a Black female who has experienced ongoing psychological, physical, and sexual violence by a Black spouse or significant other. In this instance, the Black male's gender may potentially be an obstacle to the Black woman allowing herself to be vulnerable and process painful thoughts, emotions, and experiences regarding her abuse. Ellis' (1994) ABCD model will be used to frame this example. If the Black male CBT clinician were to self-disclose a problematic issue regarding his spouse, girlfriend, or daughter (A), the Black female client may view that disclosure through a core belief that maintains men cannot be trusted or are malicious in nature (B), and consequences (C) of such a disclosure could be disdain for the Black male CBT clinician, distrust, or other emotional or behavioral outcomes which may undermine therapeutic rapport with the Black male CBT clinician. There are an infinite number of ways in which self-disclosure could be beneficial or detrimental with Black female and male clients in CBT. Constantine and Kwan (2003) have suggested that the therapist consider the reasons for the therapist's self-disclosure, the client's anticipated appreciation of or benefit from the self-disclosure, and the goals of the therapist's self-disclosure. Along those lines, in CBT the clinician self-disclosure may also be considered in terms of how the client may perceive the new information about the therapist given the client's cognitive-behavioral case conceptualization, the automatic thoughts and core beliefs of the client, the impact the new information may have on cognitive restructuring interventions, the CBT clinician's current assessment of therapeutic rapport, and the client's experiences with structural racism.

8.3 The Strong Black Woman Schema: Implications for Cognitive Restructuring and Social Support

In this book, the Strong Black Woman or Superwoman schema (Beauboeuf-Lafontant, 2008) was first discussed in Chap. 4, regarding maladaptive beliefs that are rooted in structural racism (Liao et al., 2020; Godbolt et al., 2022). The Strong Black Woman and Superwoman schemas are used interchangeably in the present text. The Strong Black Woman schema is characterized by beliefs that she should: show strength, not express emotions, not show vulnerability, succeed at all costs, and be altruistic toward others (Woods-Giscombé & Black, 2010). The Strong Black Woman schema has been empirically associated with perfectionism (Liao et al., 2020) and depression in Black women (Spivey et al., 2024). The study by Spivey and associates also found that as the Black female sample's level of belief in the Strong Black Woman schema increased, their beliefs in seeking social support decreased. Another study has shown that as Black women's beliefs in the Strong Black Woman schema increase, their perceptions of available emotional social support decreased (Watson-Singleton, 2017). The same study also found that as the women's beliefs in the Strong Black Woman schema increased, their psychological distress increased. Given the frequency with which the Strong Black Woman schema occurs and the negative emotional and behavioral consequences of the schema (Parks & Hayman, 2024), the Strong Black Woman schema is a legitimate target for cognitive restructuring with Black American women and should be included in the cognitive-behavioral case conceptualization.

In accordance with principle 6 (*Evaluating Thoughts and Beliefs*), the Strong Black Woman schema can be restructured without violating the first RESPPECTUS principle of *Resilience and Strength of Black Americans*. The first RESPPECTUS principle could be embodied via using empathic and affirming responses (principle 2: *Empathy for Black Traumatic Events and Stressors*) to the Black woman's positive qualities and experience. In essence, RESPPECTUS principles 1 and 2, would be synergistically used as they pertain to processing issues regarding Black women in CBT. In the study by Beauboeuf-Lafontant (2007) Black women indicated their desire to have their success recognized. Due to the lack of mutual exclusivity between affirming success and still needing others for support, affirmations of accomplishments can be done in CBT with Black women without buttressing the Strong Black Woman schema. However, depending on the specific Black woman a CBT clinician is working with, whether a reflection or affirmation is viewed as being supportive or endorsing the Strong Black Woman schema would ultimately be determined by the Black female client. Hence, the need to learn the unique style, attributes, and perceptions of each Black woman the clinician is working with (principle 9: *Uniqueness of Each Black Individual*). The content of what is being acknowledged and affirmed is fundamentally different from what the target of a cognitive restructuring exercise would be. Cognitive restructuring regarding the Strong Black Woman schema would identify, challenge, and modify maladaptive thoughts and beliefs pertaining to one-dimensional views of a Black woman being detrimentally selfless. The study conducted by Beauboeuf-Lafontant (2007) has discussed negative thoughts and beliefs within the Strong Black Women schema. These potentially detrimental Strong Black Woman schema cognitions include Black women viewing themselves as:

- Deficient if she needs or is using various forms of social support.
- Negative or bad if advocating for herself.
- Less than, if choosing to prioritize her own needs.
- Always having to sacrifice herself to better someone else.

The thoughts and beliefs associated with the Strong Black Woman schema may certainly be challenged using traditional CBT Socratic questions pertaining to evidence, cost–benefit analysis, and other frequently used cognitive interventions. Cognitive restructuring regarding the Strong Black Woman schema may also be effectively achieved using carefully planned behavioral experiments. The logic behind using behavioral experiments is that the experience of doing behaviors that are contrary to the Strong Black Woman schema, such as asking for help, allowing others to do for the Black woman, and self-advocacy, may aid in disconfirming the evidentiary basis and perceived utility of the Strong Black Woman schema.

Principle 10 addresses *Social Support's Import*. The role of social support becomes more complicated when viewed within the context of the Strong Black Woman schema. Although adverse circumstances immediately necessitating support from others may not always permit it, it may be clinically efficient to use behavioral interventions to begin seeking and acquiring social support once the Black woman has some substantive belief that asking for help may be beneficial or not demoralizing. Introducing behavioral interventions to secure social support before the Black female client believes such support is useful may be out of sync with the client's readiness to change. The client's cognitive-behavioral case conceptualization, research, clinical supervision, and seeking the client's feedback may be useful in determining the optimal time to begin behavioral interventions to aid the Black woman in seeking support. There are various behavioral interventions that could be used to mobilize social support for the Black woman. These behavioral interventions include, but are not limited to problem-solving, role-playing regarding asking for various forms of support and help, as well as assertiveness training. Finally, given that the Strong Black Woman schema is substantively tied to structural factors, there is also a simultaneous need for policy change (principle 5) that can address structural inequities including wages, health, and resources (Parks & Hayman, 2024).

8.4 Cognitive-Behavioral Therapy with Black Diasporic Groups

Anti-Black structural racism is not limited to the United States. The influence of anti-Black structural racism has been experienced in various geographical locations across multiple contexts. The context of this text has referred to CBT regarding anti-Black structural racism in the United States of America (USA), however the cognitive-behavioral RESPPECTUS principles also have some utility for Black individuals who experience structural racism in other parts of the world. Below notable examples of anti-Black structural racism are provided. However, this list is not exhaustive and is provided to identify other geographies and histories regarding Black African descendants, for which the cognitive-behavioral RESPPECTUS principles may be relevant.

8.4.1 North America: Canada

In the past, the author routinely did presentations on CBT with Black Americans in Canada. When discussing CBT with Black Americans, the Canadian audience discussed with the author how important it was that Black racial progress also be achieved in Canada. Within the North American continent, the US is typically identified as the importer of enslaved Africans. Many free Africans in America sought out Canada as a refuge from slavery and structural racism experienced in the United States (Reese, 2011). According to Reese, Harriet Tubman saw herself and her escape from slavery in the United States as being similar to Israelites who were fleeing slavery from Pharoah in Egypt, except Canada was viewed as the Promised Land. Despite it being traditionally associated with the underground railroad and Black liberation (McCorkindale, 2023), Canada has had Africans who were in bondage and liberated on its land for hundreds of years (Nelson, 2020). Similar to the United States, structural racism has manifested itself in various ways throughout Canadian society (Noorishad et al., 2023), laws and social policy (James, 2023), and mental healthcare (Rao, 2022). Given the history and current social landscape of Canada, the CBT RESPPECTUS principles for Black Americans may also have relevance for Black Canadians as well.

8.4.2 South Africa

The US and South Africa share many similarities as it pertains to structural racism and laws which created and sustained apartheid (Sides, 2017). Structural racism within the US has already been discussed in Chap. 2, therefore, the current section identifies ways in which the two countries overlap regarding apartheid and the potential implications of the cognitive-behavioral RESPPECTUS principles for Black South Africans. South African Apartheid, legal segregation based on race, is often compared to Jim Crow laws in the United States. Similar to the United States, South African apartheid resulted in health disparities (Bell et al., 2022), psychological and social problems that still persists in South Africa today (Harriman et al., 2022). The intertwining of structural racism and mental health care in South Africa could create some potential value for the use of the cognitive-behavioral RESPPECTUS principles when working with Black South Africans.

8.4.3 South America

It may be surprising to some to know that Brazil has received more enslaved persons than the US (Slave Voyages, 2021). However, Chile, Central America, and Mexico were countries that did not see the rampant growth of enslaved persons during the 1800s (Sobrevilla Perea, 2023). The negative health consequences are still evident in Brazil in the form of disproportionate maternal mortality (Small et al., 2017) and infant mortality (Nyarko et al., 2015) statistics among Black women and children, respectively. Similar to America, disparate mental health outcomes of Black individuals are also seen in Brazil, with Black individuals showing the least usage of primary health care and having higher mortality as it pertained to mental health disorders relative to White individuals (Medeiros et al., 2023).

Be it North America, South America, or Africa, similar patterns of slavery, structural racism, and physical and mental health disparities occur. These structural factors and their common impacts on the mental health of individuals across the Black diaspora underscore the potential utility of cognitive-behavioral principles that seek to address the varied and common impacts of structural racism. France, the Netherlands, Spain, and other geographic regions also received enslaved Africans (Slave Voyages, 2021). More detailed discussions of the international Black mental health impact of structural racism can be found elsewhere in the behavioral and social science literature.

8.4.4 The RESPPECTUS Principles and Black Diasporic Groups

While the majority of the cognitive-behavioral RESPPECTUS principles may appear fairly relevant for Black individuals regardless of country of origin, the RESPPECTUS principles may be utilized slightly differently outside of the United States. The first principle, *Resilience and Strength of Black Americans*, does not necessarily need to be geographically restricted. As discussed in Chap. 1, prior to the Transatlantic slave trade, Africans were responsible for various scientific and civic contributions to humanity (Jackson, 2017). Black individuals, be they American or otherwise, may adopt a broader collective perspective and draw strength and resilience from the common ancestral core of Black African people. This collective consideration of Black strength may also aid in countering internalized racism that may manifest as anti-Black xenophobia or demonization of other Black individuals who do not share a common country of origin. As it pertains to principle 2, *Empathy for Black Traumatic Events and Stressors*, cognitive-behavioral clinicians may be in the US but, for example, working with a Black African who has immigrated from Eritrea. While the country and historical background of an African person from Eritrea may differ from that of a Black American, the key components of Principle 2 (empathic communications about traumatic events and structural racism) remain important. Alternatively, an American cognitive-behavioral clinician working with a Black Canadian in Canada, may romantically assume that Canada is free of all structural and interpersonal racism; such an assumption could damage the therapeutic rapport with the Black Canadian client or otherwise hinder progress in CBT. Principle 5 addresses *Policy Change*. Various countries have their respective governmental processes for achieving policy change. Factors that facilitate or stifle policy changes that would be advantageous to Black individuals experiencing mental health problems would vary depending on the country and the distribution of power. The vast differences that may exist between Black individuals in America and other individuals within the Black diaspora also underscore the importance of a substantive cognitive-behavioral case conceptualization that thoroughly examines strengths as well as beliefs about and experiences with structural racism. See Chap. 5 regarding cognitive-behavioral case conceptualizations with Black Americans for additional information.

8.5 Chapter 8: Cognitive-Behavioral Therapy: Black Men, Women, & Black Diasporic Groups: Summary

The present chapter discussed the applications of the cognitive-behavioral RESPPECTUS principles to Black American men, women, and diasporic Black groups in Canada, South America, and South Africa. Important features of the present chapter included the Black American disparities, stereotypes, empathy, strengths, and social positioning of Black American men and women in the context of CBT. In the discussion of Black diasporic groups, some parallels were drawn with Black Americans in the United States.

8.6 Concluding Thoughts Regarding the Cognitive-Behavioral RESPPECTUS Principles

The cognitive-behavioral RESPPECTUS principles were based primarily on extant research as well as the clinical experience of the author in working with Black Americans in both clinical and empirical settings. Given research that undergirds the principles and the clinical logic of their application with Black Americans and others within the Black diaspora, the author anticipates that the text will aid in building rapport, constructing cognitive-behavioral case conceptualizations, applying cognitive-behavioral interventions, and overall advancement of CBT with Black Americans. The author also anticipates that the RESPPECTUS principles will be of substantive benefit to clinical researchers who study CBT with Black Americans and other individuals within the Black diaspora. The author wishes to thank the Black clients with whom the author has worked over the years and the Black research participants who helped spur some of the ideals and clarity regarding the cognitive-behavioral RESPPECTUS principles.

References

Abrams, J. A., Hill, A., & Maxwell, M. (2019). Underneath the mask of the strong black woman schema: Disentangling influences of strength and self-silencing on depressive symptoms among US black women. *Sex Roles: A Journal of Research, 80*(9–10), 517–526. https://doi.org/10.1007/s11199-018-0956-y

Alexander, M. (2010). *The new Jim crow: Mass incarceration in the ages of colorblindness*. The New Press.

Ash, M. J., Livingston, M. D., Sales, J. M., & Woods-Jaeger, B. (2024). Mental health treatment utilization and unmet mental health needs among black reproductive-age women in the United States. *Psychiatric Services*. Advance online publication. https://doi.org/10.1176/appi.ps.20230464

Basile Ibrahim, B., Barcelona, V., Condon, E. M., Crusto, C. A., & Taylor, J. Y. (2021). The association between neighborhood social vulnerability and cardiovascular health risk among black/African American women in the InterGEN study. *Nursing Research, 70*, S3–S12. https://doi.org/10.1097/NNR.0000000000000523

Beauboeuf-Lafontant, T. (2007). "You have to show strength": An exploration of gender, race, and depression. *Gender & Society, 21*(1), 28–51. https://doi.org/10.1177/0891243206294108

Beauboeuf-Lafontant, T. (2008). Listening past the lies that make us sick: A voice-centered analysis of strength and depression among black women. *Qualitative Sociology, 31*(4), 391–406. https://doi.org/10.1007/s11133-008-9113-1

Beck, J. S. (2021). *Cognitive behavior therapy: Basics and beyond* (3rd ed.). Guilford Press.

Bell, G. C., & Harris, T. M. (2017). Exploring representations of black masculinity and emasculation on NBC'S parenthood. *Journal of International and Intercultural Communication, 10*(2), 135–152. https://doi.org/10.1080/17513057.2016.1142598

Bell, G. J., Ncayiyana, J., Sholomon, A., Goel, V., Zuma, K., & Emch, M. (2022). Race place and HIV: The legacies of apartheid and racist policy in South Africa. *Social Science & Medicine, 296*(114755), 10. https://doi.org/1016/j.socscimed.2022.114755

Berger, P. L., & Luckmann, T. (1966). *The social construction of reality: A treatise in the sociology of knowledge*. Anchor Books.

Boyd, R. (2022). Racial disproportionality and disparity in child welfare: A problem with "bias" in the research. *Child Welfare, 100*(1), 29–49.

Briggs, H. E., Huggins-Hoyt, K. Y., Teasley, M. L., & Hopps, J. G. (2022). Poverty or racism?: Determinants of disproportionality and disparity for African American/black children in child welfare. *Research on Social Work Practice, 32*(5), 533–538. https://doi.org/10.1177/10497315221076830

Cadaret, M. C., & Speight, S. L. (2018). An exploratory study of attitudes toward psychological help seeking among African American men. *Journal of Black Psychology, 44*(4), 347–370. https://doi.org/10.1177/0095798418774655

Cecil, D. K. (2024). Saying her name: Gendered narratives in news coverage of Breonna Taylor's death. *Race and Justice, 14*(3), 423–439. https://doi.org/10.1177/21533687211070552

Center for Behavioral Health Statistics and Quality. (2021). *Racial/ethnic differences in mental health service use among adults and adolescents (2015-2019)* (publication no. PEP21–07–01-002). Substance Abuse and Mental Health Services Administration. Retrieved from https://www.samhsa.gov/data/

Centers for Disease Control and Prevention. (2024, January 17). *Health disparities in Black or African American people*. https://www.cdc.gov/health-disparities-hiv-std-tb-hepatitis/populations/black-african-american.html?CDC_AAref_Val=https://www.cdc.gov/nchhstp/healthdisparities/africanamericans.html

Chung, B., Meldrum, M., Jones, F., Brown, A., & Jones, L. (2014). Perceived sources of stress and resilience in men in an African American community. *Progress in Community Health Partnerships: Research, Education, and Action, 8*(4), 441–451. https://doi.org/10.1353/cpr.2014.0053

Coates, E. E., Moore, C., de Brumley, H. R. C., Prudhomme, A., Edwards, L., & Curtis, L. (2024). Black mothers' ethnic–racial socialization one year after highly publicized anti-black murders during the pandemic. *Journal of Research on Adolescence, 34*(3), 831–844. https://doi.org/10.1111/jora.12948

Constantine, M. G., & Kwan, K.-L. K. (2003). Cross-cultural considerations of therapist self-disclosure. *Journal of Clinical Psychology, 59*(5), 581–588. https://doi-org.proxy.ulib.uits.iu.edu/10.1002/jclp.10160

Davis, S. M. (2018). Taking back the power: An analysis of black women's communicative resistance. *Review of Communication, 18*(4), 301–318. https://doi.org/10.1080/15358593.2018.1461234

Earl, T. R., Alegría, M., Mendieta, F., & Linhart, Y. D. (2011). "just be straight with me:" an exploration of black patient experiences in initial mental health encounters. *The American Journal of Orthopsychiatry, 81*(4), 519–525. https://doi.org/10.1111/j.1939-0025.2011.01123.x

Edwards, F., Lee, H., & Esposito, M. (2019). Risk of being killed by police use of force in the United States by age, race-ethnicity, and sex. *Proceedings of the National Academy of Sciences of the United States of America, 116*(34), 16793–16798. https://doi.org/10.1073/pnas.1821204116

Egan, G., & Reese, R. J. (2019). *The skilled helper: A problem-management & opportunity-development approach to helping* (11th ed.). Cengage.

Eldridge, L., & Berrigan, D. (2022). Structural racism and triple-negative breast cancer among black and white women in the United States. *Health Equity, 6*(1), 116–123. https://doi.org/10.1089/heq.2021.0041

Ellis, A. (1994). *Reason and emotion in psychotherapy: A comprehensive method of treating human disturbances (Revised and updated)*. Carol Publishing Group.

Godbolt, D., Opara, I., & Amutah-Onukagha, N. (2022). Strong Black Women: Linking stereotypes, stress, and overeating among a sample of Black female college students. *Journal of Black Studies, 53*(6), 609–634. https://doi.org/10.1177/00219347221087453

Gregory, V. L., Jr., & Clary, K. L. (2022). Addressing anti-black racism: The roles of social work. *Smith College Studies In Social Work, 92*(1), 1–27. https://doi.org/10.1080/00377317.2021.2008287

Gregory, V. L., Jr., & Tucker Edmonds, J. L. (2023). The racial pandemic experienced by black American men: Cognitive-behavioral and structural implications. *American Journal of Orthopsychiatry, 93*(1), 1–16. https://doi.org/10.1037/ort0000651

Gregory, V. L., Jr., & Tucker Edmonds, J. L. (2024a). Cultural trauma scale: Psychometric evaluation of black men's beliefs, emotions, and coping. *Psychological Trauma: Theory, Research, Practice, and Policy, 16*(8), 1329–1337. https://doi.org/10.1037/tra0001607

Gregory, V. L., Jr., & Tucker Edmonds, J. L. (2024b). Cultural trauma scale (CuTS): Parsimonious principal component analysis, independent black American male sample. *Journal of Aggression, Maltreatment & Trauma, 33*(3), 369–386. https://doi.org/10.1080/10926771.2023.2256741

Gregory, V. L., Jr., Miller, B., & L., & Lipsey, A. (in press). Black men, structural racism, cultural barriers: Structural equation model with cognitive-behavioral implications. *The Counseling Psychologist.*

Guglielminotti, J., Samari, G., Friedman, A. M., Landau, R., & Li, G. (2024). State-level indicators of structural racism and severe adverse maternal outcomes during childbirth. *Maternal & Child Health Journal, 28*(1), 165–176. https://doi.org/10.1007/s10995-023-03828-9

Hankerson, S. H., Suite, D., & Bailey, R. K. (2015). Treatment disparities among African American men with depression: Implications for clinical practice. *Journal of Health Care for the Poor and Underserved, 26*(1), 21–34. https://doi.org/10.1353/hpu.2015.0012

Harriman, N. W., Williams, D. R., Morgan, J. W., Sewpaul, R., Manyaapelo, T., Sifunda, S., Mabaso, M., Mbewu, A. D., & Reddy, S. P. (2022). Racial disparities in psychological distress in post-apartheid South Africa: Results from the SANHANES-1 survey. *Social Psychiatry and Psychiatric Epidemiology: The International Journal for Research in Social and Genetic Epidemiology and Mental Health Services, 57*(4), 843–857. https://doi.org/10.1007/s00127-021-02175-w

Holdsworth, E., Bowen, E., Brown, S., Howat, D. (2014). Client engagement in psychotherapeutic treatment and associations with client characteristics therapist characteristics and treatment factors. *Clinical Psychology Review, 34*(5), 428–450. https://doi.org/10.1016/j.cpr.2014.06.004

Huey, S. J., Jr., Park, A. L., Galán, C. A., & Wang, C. X. (2023). Culturally responsive cognitive behavioral therapy for ethnically diverse populations. *Annual Review of Clinical Psychology, 19*, 51–78. https://doi.org/10.1146/annurev-clinpsy-080921-072750

Jackson, J. G. (2017). *Ethiopia and the origin of civilization*. African Studies African Tree Press.

James, C. E. (2023). Who gets to be "Canadian"? How race has operated in keeping Canada white. *Journal of Canadian Studies, 57*(3), 317–338. https://doi.org/10.3138/jcs-2023-0035

Joseph, J. (2022). Invisible police lethal violence against black women in the United States: An intersectional approach. *Peace Review, 34*(2), 177–186. https://doi.org/10.1080/10402659.2022.2044729

Kahneman, D. (2011). *Thinking, fast and slow*. Farrar, Straus, and Giroux.

Leahy, R. (1996). *Cognitive therapy: Basic principles and applications*. Jason Aronson.

Leath, S., Billingsley, J., Jones, M., Johnson, K., Taliaferro, J., & Gaskin-Cole, G. (2023). Raising resilient black women: A study of superwoman mothering and strength as a form of gendered racial socialization in black mother-daughter relationships. *Sex Roles: A Journal of Research, 89*(11–12), 625–642. https://doi.org/10.1007/s11199-023-01417-2

Liao, K. Y.-H., Wei, M., & Yin, M. (2020). The misunderstood schema of the strong black woman: Exploring its mental health consequences and coping responses among African American women. *Psychology of Women Quarterly, 44*(1), 84–104. https://doi.org/10.1177/0361684319883198

McCorkindale, D. (2023). Weaponized history: The underground railroad's mythologized legacy in Canada. *American Review of Canadian Studies, 53*(1), 68–81. https://doi.org/10.1080/02722011.2023.2172886

Medeiros, S., Coelho, R., Millett, C., Saraceni, V., Coeli, C. M., Trajman, A., Rasella, D., Durovni, B., & Hone, T. (2023). Racial inequalities in mental healthcare use and mortality: A cross-sectional analysis of 1.2 million low-income individuals in Rio de Janeiro, Brazil 2010-2016. *BMJ Global Health, 8*(12), e013327.

Mehra, R., Alspaugh, A., Franck, L. S., McLemore, M. R., Kershaw, T. S., Ickovics, J. R., Keene, D. E., & Sewell, A. A. (2022). "Police shootings, now that seems to be the main issue"—black pregnant women's anticipation of police brutality towards their children. *BMC Public Health, 22*(1), 1–8. https://doi.org/10.1186/s12889-022-12557-7

Miller, W. R., & Rollnick, S. (2023). *Motivational interviewing: Helping people change and grow* (4th ed.). Guilford Press.

Motley, R., & Banks, A. (2018). Black males, trauma, and mental health service use: A Systematic Review. *Perspectives on Social Work, 14*(1), 4–19.

Nelson, C. A. (2020). A "tone of voice peculiar to new-England": Fugitive slave advertisements and the heterogeneity of enslaved people of African descent in eighteenth-century Quebec. *Current Anthropology, 61*(S22), S304–S316. https://doi-org.proxy.ulib.uits.iu.edu/10.1086/709976

Noorishad, P.-G., Paul Darius, W., Czechowski, K., McIntee, S.-E., Ntunga Mukunzi, J., & Mary Cénat, J. (2023). Racism as a vehicle for the overrepresentation of black youth in child protection services in Ontario, Canada: Caseworkers' and community facilitators' perspectives. *Children and Youth Services Review, 149*, 1–10. https://doi.org/10.1016/j.childyouth.2023.106963

Nyarko, K. A., Lopez-Camelo, J., Castilla, E. E., & Wehby, G. L. (2015). Explaining racial disparities in infant health in Brazil. *American Journal of Public Health, 105*(Suppl 4), S575. https://doi.org/10.2105/AJPH.2012.301021r

Okoro, O. N., Nelson, C. S., Witherspoon, S. P., Witherspoon, S. F., & Simmons, G. E., Jr. (2020). Culturally responsive health promotion to address health disparities in African American men: A program impact evaluation. *American Journal of Men's Health, 14*(4). https://doi.org/10.1177/1557988320951321

Parks, A. K., & Hayman, L. L. (2024). Unveiling the strong black woman schema—evolution and impact: A systematic review. *Clinical Nursing Research, 33*(5), 395–404. https://doi.org/10.1177/10547738241234425

Randolph, S. D., Golin, C., Welgus, H., Lightfoot, A. F., Harding, C. J., & Riggins, L. F. (2020). How perceived structural racism and discrimination and medical mistrust in the health system influences participation in HIV health services for black women living in the United States south: A qualitative, descriptive study. *JANAC Journal of the Association of Nurses in AIDS Care, 31*(5), 598–605. https://doi.org/10.1097/JNC.0000000000000189

Rao, S. (2022). Black lives, blue shirts and 'colourblindness': Application of critical race theory in police response models for persons with mental illness. *Community Mental Health Journal, 58*(1), 1–10. https://doi.org/10.1007/s10597-021-00888-5

Reese, R. (2011). Canada: The promised land for U.S. Slaves. *Western Journal of Black Studies, 35*(3), 208–217.

Rogers, C. R. (1957). The necessary and sufficient conditions of therapeutic personality change. *Journal of Consulting Psychology, 21*(2), 95–103. https://doi.org/10.1037/h0045357

Sangamon County Illinois. (2024). *Sonya Massey information*. https://sangamonil.gov/departments/s-z/sheriff/sonya-massey-information

Sharpless, L., Kershaw, T., Knight, D., Campbell, J. K., Phillips, K., Katague, M., & Willie, T. C. (2024). Moving towards transformative justice for black women survivors of intimate partner violence: An intersectional qualitative study. *BMC Public Health, 24*(1), 2730. https://doi.org/10.1186/s12889-024-20244-y

Shannon, J. (2023). A study of help-seeking behaviors for African American men: Implications for counselor education. *Journal of Multicultural Counseling & Development, 51*(3), 183–194. https://doi.org/10.1002/jmcd.12275

Shea, M., Wong, Y. J., Nguyen, K. K., & Gonzalez, P. D. (2019). College students' barriers to seeking mental health counseling: Scale development and psychometric evaluation. *Journal of Counseling Psychology, 66*(5), 626–639. https://doi.org/10.1037/cou0000356

Sheehy, S., Brock, M., Palmer, J. R., Albert, M. A., Cozier, Y. C., & Rosenberg, L. (2024). Perceived interpersonal racism in relation to incident coronary heart disease among black women. *Circulation, 149*(7), 521–528. https://doi.org/10.1161/CIRCULATIONAHA.123.066471

Shim, R. S. (2021). Dismantling structural racism in psychiatry: A path to mental health equity. *American Journal of Psychiatry, 178*(7), 592–598. https://doi.org/10.1176/appi.ajp.2021.21060558

Sides, K. B. (2017). Precedence and warning: Global apartheid and South Africa's long conversation on race with the United States. *Safundi, 18*(3), 221–238. https://doi.org/10.1080/17533171.2017.1324081

Slave Voyages. (2021). *Trans-Atlantic slave trade—Estimates*. https://www.slavevoyages.org/assessment/estimates

Small, M. J., Allen, T. K., & Brown, H. L. (2017). Global disparities in maternal morbidity and mortality. *Seminars in Perinatology, 41*(5), 318–322. https://doi.org/10.1053/j.semperi.2017.04.009

Smith, C. A. (2021). Impossible privacy: Black women and police terror. *Black Scholar, 51*(1), 20–29. https://doi.org/10.1080/00064246.2020.1855090

Smith, D. Y., & Roane, A. (2023). Child removal fears and black mothers' medical decision-making. *Contexts: Understanding People in Their Social Worlds, 22*(1), 18–23. https://doi.org/10.1177/15365042221142834

Sobrevilla Perea, N. (2023). The abolition of slavery in the south American republics. *Slavery & Abolition, 44*(1), 90–108. https://doi.org/10.1080/0144039X.2022.2122814

Spivey, B. N., Abrams, J. A., Watson-Singleton, N. N., & Metzger, I. W. (2024). "I can do bad all by myself": Indirect effect of social support beliefs on the strong black woman schema and depressive symptoms. *Cultural Diversity & Ethnic Minority Psychology*. https://doi.org/10.1037/cdp0000672

Subica, A. M., & Link, B. G. (2022). Cultural trauma as a fundamental cause of health disparities. *Social Science & Medicine, 292*. https://doi.org/10.1016/j.socscimed.2021.114574

Talbert, R. D. (2023). Lethal police encounters and cardiovascular health among black Americans. *Journal of Racial and Ethnic Health Disparities, 10*(4), 1756–1767. https://doi.org/10.1007/s40615-022-01359-7

Taylor, E., Guy-Walls, P., Wilkerson, P., & Addae, R. (2019). The historical perspectives of stereotypes on African-American males. *Journal of Human Rights and Social Work, 4*, 213–225. https://doi.org/10.1007/s41134-019-00096-y

Teti, M., Martin, A. E., Ranade, R., Massie, J., Malebranche, D. J., Tschann, J. M., & Bowleg, L. (2012). "I'm a keep rising. I'm a keep going forward, regardless": Exploring black men's resilience amid sociostructural challenges and stressors. *Qualitative Health Research, 22*(4), 524–533. https://doi.org/10.1177/1049732311422051

Thomas Tobin, C. S., Gutiérrez, Á., Erving, C. L., Norris, K. C., & Thorpe, R. J., Jr. (2022). When resilience becomes risk: A latent class analysis of psychosocial resources and allostatic load among African American men. *American Journal of Men's Health, 16*(3). https://doi.org/10.1177/15579883221104272

Vontress, C. E. (1971). Racial differences: Impediments to rapport. *Journal of Counseling Psychology, 18*(1), 7–13. https://doi.org/10.1037/h0030758

Ward, E. C., Wiltshire, J. C., Detry, M. A., & Brown, R. L. (2013). African American men and women's attitude toward mental illness, perceptions of stigma, and preferred coping behaviors. *Nursing Research, 62*(3), 185–194. https://doi.org/10.1097/NNR.0b013e31827bf533

Watson-Singleton, N. N. (2017). Strong black woman schema and psychological distress: The mediating role of perceived emotional support. *Journal of Black Psychology, 43*(8), 778–788. https://doi.org/10.1177/0095798417732414

West, L. M., Donovan, R. A., & Daniel, A. R. (2016). The price of strength: Black college women's perspectives on the strong black woman stereotype. *Women & Therapy, 39*(3–4), 390–412. https://doi.org/10.1080/02703149.2016.1116871

Willingham, B. (2018). Black women and state violence: A history of victimization and exclusion. *Canadian Review of American Studies, 48*(1), 77–94. https://doi.org/10.3138/cras.2017.018

Williams, S. (2021). Stream of sadness: Young black women's racial trauma, police brutality and social media. *Feminist Media Studies, 21*(8), 1270–1284. https://doi.org/10.1080/14680777.2021.2006261

Woods-Giscombé, C. L., & Black, A. R. (2010). Mind-body interventions to reduce risk for health disparities related to stress and strength among African American Women: The potential of mindfulness-based stress reduction loving-kindness and the NTU therapeutic framework. *Complementary Health Practice Review, 15*(3), 115–131. https://doi.org/10.1177/1533210110386776

Woods-Giscombe, C. L., Williams, K. P., Conklin, J., Dodd, A., Bravo, L., Anderson, A. M., Frazier, T., Bey, G., Robinson, M. N., Warren, B. J., Wight, K. D., Felix, A. S., Anderson, C. M., & Hood, D. B. (2023). A scoping review of the concept of resilience among African American women. *Archives of Psychiatric Nursing, 46*, 107–120. https://doi.org/10.1016/j.apnu.2023.04.008

Appendix A: Cognitive-Behavioral Therapy with Black Americans: Clinical Research

Throughout this text, the tendency to integrate the findings of cognitive-behavioral interventions of Black Americans with other racial and ethnic minority groups has been described. The summarization of Black and other racial and ethnic minority research makes sense if the goal of integrating the findings is to collectively describe cognitive-behavioral outcomes of racial and ethnic minorities overall. However, clinicians who primarily work with Black Americans using CBT may have clinically relevant research questions that remain largely unanswered. A list of empirical studies evaluating second-wave CBT for various mental and physical health conditions is provided below. The list is provided as an additional resource to those clinicians who may not have access to formal electronic databases. Medline was searched with the phrase "Cognitive-behavioral therapy and Black" (February 2025); this search yielded 488 references. To be included in the list of cognitive-behavioral empirical studies references had: (1) Participants whom were Black (one or both arms of the studies with at least 90% Black individuals receiving CBT) or reviews or meta-analyses were specific to Black individuals, (2) the intervention must have included a second-wave cognitive-behavioral therapy with some form of cognitive restructuring, (3) individual clinical trials could include one-group pretest-posttest, quasi-experimental trials, or randomized controlled trials. The title and abstracts of references were read to determine if the reference met inclusion criteria. The references of included studies were inspected for other studies, which may meet inclusion criteria. Cognitive-behavioral studies meeting inclusion criteria, which were previously citied in this text, were also included in the list below. The following list involving Black participants also includes empirical trials the author was aware of but that were not documented in the review of Medline. The list is not exhaustive. Given the overlap in outcomes within studies and the use of various CBT modalities, the references for each diagnostic or modality category are not necessarily mutually exclusive.

V. L. Gregory, Jr., *Cognitive-Behavioral Therapy with Black Americans*,
https://doi.org/10.1007/978-3-032-01666-9

Bibliography

Anxiety

Bouwer, C., & Stein, D. J. (1998). Survivors of torture presenting at an anxiety disorders clinic: Symptomatology and pharmacotherapy. *Journal of Nervous and Mental Disease, 186*(5), 316–318. https://doi.org/10.1097/00005053-199805000-00009

Bonilla-Escobar, F. J., Fandiño-Losada, A., Martínez-Buitrago, D. M., Santaella-Tenorio, J., Tobón-García, D., Muñoz-Morales, E. J., Escobar-Roldán, I. D., Babcock, L., Duarte-Davidson, E., Bass, J. K., Murray, L. K., Dorsey, S., Gutierrez-Martinez, M. I., & Bolton, P. (2018). A randomized controlled trial of a transdiagnostic cognitive-behavioral intervention for Afro-descendants' survivors of systemic violence in Colombia. *PLoS One, 13*(12), e0208483. https://doi.org/10.1371/journal.pone.0208483

Carter, M. M., Sbrocco, T., Gore, K. L., Marin, N. W., & Lewis, E. L. (2003). Cognitive–behavioral group therapy versus a wait-list control in the treatment of African American women with panic disorder. *Cognitive Therapy and Research, 27*(5), 505. https://doi.org/10.1023/A:1026350903639

Chambliss, D. L., & Williams, K. E. (1995). A preliminary study of African Americans with agoraphobia: Symptom severity and outcome of treatment with in vivo exposure. *Behavior Therapy, 26*(3), 501–515. https://doi.org/10.1016/S0005-7894(05)80097-8

Friedman, S., Braunstein, J. W., & Halpern, B. (2006). Cognitive behavioral treatment of panic disorder and agoraphobia in a multiethnic urban outpatient clinic: Initial presentation and treatment outcome. *Cognitive and Behavioral Practice, 13*(4), 282–292. https://doi.org/10.1016/j.cbpra.2006.04.009

Gregory, V. L., Jr. (2019). Cognitive-behavioral therapy for anxious symptoms in persons of African descent: A meta-Analysis. *Journal of Social Service Research, 45*(1), 87–101. https://doi.org/10.1080/01488376.2018.1479344

Holliday, R. P., Holder, N. D., Williamson, M. L. C., & Surís, A. (2017). Therapeutic response to Cognitive Processing Therapy in White and Black female veterans with military sexual trauma-related PTSD. *Cognitive Behaviour Therapy, 46*(5), 432–446. https://doi.org/10.1080/16506073.2017.1312511

Jonassaint, C. R., Gibbs, P., Belnap, B. H., Karp, J. F., Abebe, K. Z., & Rollman, B. L. (2017). Engagement and outcomes for a computerised cognitive-behavioural therapy intervention for anxiety and depression in African Americans. *BJPsych Open, 3*(1), 1–5. https://doi.org/10.1192/bjpo.bp.116.003657

Lester, K., Artz, C., & Resick, P. A. (2010). Impact of race on early treatment termination and outcomes in posttraumatic stress disorder treatment. *Journal of Consulting and Clinical Psychology, 78*(4), 480–489. https://doi.org/10.1037/a0019551

Markell, H. M., Newman, M. G., Gallop, R., Gibbons, M. B., Rickels, K., & Crits-Christoph, P. (2014). Combined medication and CBT for generalized anxiety disorder with African American participants: reliability and validity of assessments and preliminary outcomes. *Behavior therapy, 45*(4), 495–506. https://doi.org/10.1016/j.beth.2014.02.008

McMullen, J., O'Callaghan, P., Shannon, C., Black, A., & Eakin, J. (2013). Group trauma-focused cognitive-behavioural therapy with former child soldiers and other war-affected boys in the DR Congo: a randomised controlled trial. *Journal of Child Psychology and Psychiatry, and Allied Disciplines, 54*(11), 1231–1241. https://doi.org/10.1111/jcpp.12094

Neuner, F., Schauer, M., & Klaschik, C. (2004). A comparison of narrative exposure therapy, supportive counseling, and psychoeducation for treating posttraumatic stress disorder in an african refugee settlement. *Journal of Consulting and Clinical Psychology, 72*(4), 579–587. https://www.apa.org/journals

Zoellner, L. A., Feeny, N. C., Fitzgibbons, L. A., & Foa, E. B. (1999). Response of African American and caucasian women to cognitive behavioral therapy for PTSD. *Behavior Therapy, 30*(4), 581–595. https://doi.org/10.1016/S0005-7894(99)80026-4

Children and Adolescents

Annesi, J. J., Smith, A. E., & Tennant, G. (2013). Cognitive-behavioural physical activity treatment in African-American pre-schoolers: Effects of age, sex, and BMI. *Journal of Paediatrics and Child Health, 49*(2), E128–E132. https://doi.org/10.1111/jpc.12082

Bella, A. T., Ani, C., Ajuwon, A., & Omigbodun, O. (2016). Effectiveness of brief school-based, group cognitive behavioural therapy for depressed adolescents in south west Nigeria. *Child and Adolescent Mental Health, 21*(1), 44–50. https://doi.org/10.1111/camh.12104

Cooley-Strickland, M. R., Griffin, R. S., Darney, D., Otte, K., & Ko, J. (2011). Urban African American youth exposed to community violence: a school-based anxiety preventive intervention efficacy study. *Journal of Prevention and Intervention in the Community, 39*(2), 149–166. https://doi.org/10.1080/10852352.2011.556573

Ginsburg, G. S., & Drake, K. L. (2002). School-based treatment for anxious African-American adolescents: A controlled pilot study. *Journal of the American Academy of Child and Adolescent Psychiatry, 41*(7), 768–775. https://doi.org/10.1097/00004583-200207000-00007

Gordon-Hollingsworth, A. T., Becker, E. M., Ginsburg, G. S., Keeton, C., Compton, S. N., Birmaher, B. B., Sakolsky, D. J., Piacentini, J., Albano, A. M., Kendall, P. C., Suveg, C. M., & March, J. S. (2015). Anxiety disorders in Caucasian and African American children: A comparison of clinical characteristics, treatment process variables, and treatment outcomes. *Child Psychiatry and Human Development, 46*(5), 643–655. https://doi.org/10.1007/s10578-014-0507-x

Lochman, J. E., Nelson, W. M., & Sims, J. P. (1981). A cognitive behavioral program for use with aggressive children. *Journal of Clinical Child Psychology, 10*(3), 146–148. https://doi.org/10.1080/15374418109533036

O'Callaghan, P., McMullen, J., Shannon, C., Rafferty, H., & Black, A. (2013). A randomized controlled trial of trauma-focused cognitive behavioral therapy for sexually exploited, war-affected congolese girls. *Journal of the American Academy of Child and Adolescent Psychiatry, 52*(4), 359–369. https://doi.org/10.1016/j.jaac.2013.01.013

Montgomery, L., Petry, N. M., & Carroll, K. M. (2012). Moderating effects of race in clinical trial participation and outcomes among marijuana-dependent young adults. *Drug and Alcohol Dependence, 126*(3), 333–339. https://doi.org/10.1016/j.drugalcdep.2012.05.033

Stewart, R. W., Orengo-Aguayo, R., Wallace, M., Metzger, I. W., & Rheingold, A. A. (2021). Leveraging technology and cultural adaptations to increase access and engagement among trauma-exposed African American youth: Exploratory study of school-based telehealth delivery of trauma-focused cognitive behavioral therapy. *Journal of Interpersonal Violence, 36*(15/16), 7090–7109. https://doi.org/10.1177/0886260519831380

Wilson, C. J., & Cottone, R. R. (2013). Using cognitive behavior therapy in clinical work with African American children and adolescents: A Review of the Literature. *Journal of Multicultural Counseling and Development, 41*(3), 130–143. https://doi.org/10.1002/j.2161-1912.2013.00032.x

Cognitive Impairment

Owen, A., Brown, B., Deragon, K., Gottstein, E., Odman, S., Owens, R., Ozbardakci, E., Watson-Singleton, N. N., & Kulshreshtha, A. (2022). Developing an integrated cognitive behavioral therapy and motivational interviewing intervention for African Americans with mild cognitive impairment: A pilot study. *Practice Innovations, 7*(3), 241–254. https://doi.org/10.1037/pri0000182

Correctional

Spiropoulos, G. V., Van Voorhis, P., & Salisbury, E. J. (2018). Programmatic moderators of CBT correctional treatment for Whites and African Americans. *International Journal of Offender Therapy and Comparative Criminology, 62*(8), 2236–2258. https://doi.org/10.1177/0306624X17721523

Depression

Afuwape, S. A., Craig, T. K. J., Harris, T., Clarke, M., Flood, A., Olajide, D., Cole, E., Leese, M., McCrone, P., & Thornicroft, G. (2010). The Cares of Life Project (CoLP): An exploratory randomised controlled trial of a community-based intervention for Black people with common mental disorder. *Journal of Affective Disorders, 127*(1–3), 370–374. https://doi.org/10.1016/j.jad.2010.05.017

Bowe, W. (2013). *Refinement and pilot testing of a culturally enhanced treatment for depressed African Americans*. [Doctoral thesis]. University of Wisconsin-Milwaukee. https://dc.uwm.edu/etd/229

Glueckauf, R. L., Davis, W. S., Willis, F., Sharma, D., Gustafson, D. J., Hayes, J., Stutzman, M., Proctor, J., Kazmer, M. M., Murray, L., Shipman, J., McIntyre, V., Wesley, L., Schettini, G., Xu, J., Parfitt, F., Graff-Radford, N., Baxter, C., Burnett, K., et al. (2012). Telephone-based, cognitive-behavioral therapy for African American dementia caregivers with depression: Initial findings. *Rehabilitation Psychology, 57*(2), 124–139. https://doi.org/10.1037/a0028688

Gregory, V. L., Jr. (2016). Cognitive-behavioral therapy for depressive symptoms in persons of African descent: A meta-analysis. *Journal of Social Service Research, 42*(1), 113–129. https://doi.org/10.1080/01488376.2015.1084973

Himelhoch, S., Mohr, D., Maxfield, J., Clayton, S., Weber, E., Medoff, D., & Dixon, L. (2011). Feasibility of telephone-based cognitive behavioral therapy targeting major depression among urban dwelling African-American people with co-occurring HIV. *Psychology, Health and Medicine, 16*(2), 156–165. https://doi.org/10.1080/13548506.2010.534641

Kohn, L. P., Oden, T., Muñoz, R. F., Robinson, A., & Leavitt, D. (2002). Adapted cognitive behavioral group therapy for depressed low-income African American women. *Community Mental Health Journal, 38*(6), 497–504. https://doi.org/10.1023/a:1020884202677

Markowitz, J. C., Spielman, L. A., Sullivan, M., & Fishman, B. (2000). An exploratory study of ethnicity and psychotherapy outcome among HIV-positive patients with depressive symptoms. *Journal of Psychotherapy Practice and Research, 9*(4), 226–231.

Meng, H., Marino, V. R., Conner, K. O., Sharma, D., Davis, W. S., & Glueckauf, R. L. (2021). Effects of in-person and telephone-based cognitive behavioral therapies on health services use and expenditures among African-American dementia caregivers with depressive symptoms. *Ethnicity and Health, 26*(6), 879–892. https://doi.org/10.1080/13557858.2019.1590536

Mynatt, S., Wicks, M., & Bolden, L. (2008). Pilot study of INSIGHT therapy in African American women. *Archives of Psychiatric Nursing, 22*(6), 364–374. https://doi.org/10.1016/j.apnu.2007.10.007

Napholz, L. (2005). An effectiveness trial to increase psychological well-being and reduce stress among African American Blue-Collar Working Women. In K. V. Oxington (Ed.), *Psychology of stress* (pp. 17–33). Nova Biomedical Books.

Ward, E. C., & Brown, R. L. (2015). A culturally adapted depression intervention for African American adults experiencing depression: Oh, happy day. *American Journal of Orthopsychiatry, 85*, 11–22. https://doi.org/10.1037/ort0000027

Group Therapy

Ali, K. M. (2008). The effects of two marathon group therapy interventions on the levels of depression and state anxiety in African American women infected with HIV/AIDS Doctoral dissertation. Retrieved from PsycINFO (3331071).

Jones, L. V., & Warner, L. A. (2011). Evaluating culturally responsive group work with black women. *Research on Social Work Practice, 21*(6), 737–746. https://doi.org/10.1177/1049731511411488

Kunorubwe, T. (2023). Cultural adaptations of group CBT for depressed clients from diverse backgrounds: A systematic review. *The Cognitive Behaviour Therapist, 16*, Article e35. doi: https://doi.org/10.1017/S1754470X23000302

Insomnia

Kalmbach, D. A., Cheng, P., Reffi, A. N., Seymour, G. M., Ruprich, M. K., Bazan, L. F., Pitts, D. S., Walch, O., & Drake, C. L. (2023). Racial disparities in treatment engagement and outcomes in digital cognitive behavioral therapy for insomnia among pregnant women. *Sleep Health, 9*(1), 18–25. https://doi.org/10.1016/j.sleh.2022.10.010

Liou, K. T., Garland, S. N., Meghani, S. H., Kaye, N. M., Thompson, E., Li, Q. S., & Mao, J. J. (2024). Racial differences in treatment adherence and response to acupuncture and cognitive behavioral therapy for insomnia among Black and White cancer survivors. *Cancer Medicine, 13*(16), e7344. https://doi.org/10.1002/cam4.7344

Zhou, E. S., Ritterband, L. M., Bethea, T. N., Robles, Y. P., Heeren, T. C., & Rosenberg, L. (2022). Effect of culturally tailored, internet-delivered cognitive behavioral therapy for Insomnia in Black Women: A randomized clinical trial. *JAMA Psychiatry, 79*(6), 538–549. https://doi.org/10.1001/jamapsychiatry.2022.0653

Physical Health

Andersen, L. S., Magidson, J. F., O'Cleirigh, C., Remmert, J. E., Kagee, A., Leaver, M., Stein, D. J., Safren, S. A., & Joska, J. (2018). A pilot study of a nurse-delivered cognitive behavioral therapy intervention (Ziphamandla) for adherence and depression in HIV in South Africa. *Journal of Health Psychology, 23*(6), 776–787. https://doi.org/10.1177/1359105316643375

Bogart, L. M., Dale, S. K., Daffin, G. K., Patel, K. N., Klein, D. J., Mayer, K. H., & Pantalone, D. W. (2018). Pilot intervention for discrimination-related coping among HIV-positive Black sexual minority men. *Cultural Diversity and Ethnic Minority Psychology, 24*(4), 541–551. https://doi.org/10.1037/cdp0000205

Dale, S. K., Wright, I. A., Madhu, A., Reid, R., Shahid, N. N., Wright, M., Sanders, J., Phillips, A., Rodriguez, A., & Safren, S. A. (2024). A pilot randomized control trial of the Striving Towards EmPowerment and Medication Adherence (STEP-AD) intervention for black women living with HIV. *AIDS and Behavior, 28*(10), 3483–3497. https://doi.org/10.1007/s10461-024-04408-w

Daniels, S. (2015). Cognitive behavioral therapy in patients with sickle cell disease. *Creative Nursing, 21*(1), 38–46. https://doi.org/10.1891/1078-4535.21.1.38

El-Mohandes, A. A. E., Kiely, M., Joseph, J. G., Subramanian, S., Johnson, A. A., Blake, S. M., Gantz, M. G., & El-Khorazaty, M. N. (2008). An intervention to improve postpartum outcomes in African-American mothers: a randomized controlled trial. *Obstetrics and Gynecology, 112*(3), 611–620. https://doi.org/10.1097/AOG.0b013e3181834b10

Gil, K. M., Wilson, J. J., Edens, J. L., Webster, D. A., Abrams, M. A., Orringer, E., Grant, M., Clark, W. C., & Janal, M. N. (1996). Effects of cognitive coping skills training on coping strategies and experimental pain sensitivity in African American adults with sickle cell disease. *Health Psychology: Official Journal of the Division of Health Psychology, American Psychological Association, 15*(1), 3–10. https://doi.org/10.1037/0278-6133.15.1.3

Goode, R. W., Kalarchian, M. A., Craighead, L., Conroy, M. B., Wallace, J., Jr., Eack, S. M., & Burke, L. E. (2018). The feasibility of a binge eating intervention in Black women with obesity. *Eating Behaviors, 29*, 83–90. https://doi.org/10.1016/j.eatbeh.2018.03.005

Ingman, T., Ali, S., Bhui, K., & Chalder, T. (2016). Chronic fatigue syndrome: comparing outcomes in White British and Black and minority ethnic patients after cognitive-behavioural therapy. *British Journal of Psychiatry, 209*(3), 251–256. https://doi.org/10.1192/bjp.bp.115.169300

Jonassaint, C. R., Lalama, C. M., Carroll, C. P., Badawy, S. M., Hamm, M. E., Stinson, J. N., Lalloo, C., Saraf, S. L., Gordeuk, V. R., Cronin, R. M., Shah, N., Lanzkron, S. M., Liles, D., O'Brien, J. A., Trimnell, C., Bailey, L., Lawrence, R. H., Saint Jean, L., DeBaun, M., et al. (2024). Digital cognitive behavioral therapy vs education for pain in adults with sickle cell disease. *Blood Advances, 8*(24), 6257–6266. https://doi.org/10.1182/bloodadvances.2024013861

Junkins, A., Psaros, C., Ott, C., Azuero, A., Lambert, C. C., Cropsey, K., Savage, R., Haberer, J. E., Safren, S. A., & Kempf, M.-C. (2021). Feasibility, acceptability, and preliminary impact of telemedicine-administered cognitive behavioral therapy for adherence and depression among African American women living with HIV in the rural South. *Journal of Health Psychology, 26*(14), 2730–2742. https://doi.org/10.1177/1359105320926526

Kalichman, S. C., Rompa, D., & Coley, B. (1997). Lack of positive outcomes from a cognitive-behavioral HIV and AIDS prevention intervention for inner-city men: lessons from a controlled pilot study. *AIDS Education and Prevention: Official Publication of the International Society for AIDS Education, 9*(4), 299–313.

Lechner, S. C., Whitehead, N. E., Vargas, S., Annane, D. W., Robertson, B. R., Carver, C. S., Kobetz, E., & Antoni, M. H. (2014). Does a community-based stress management intervention affect psychological adaptation among underserved black breast cancer survivors? *Journal of the National Cancer Institute Monographs, 2014*(50), 315–322. https://doi.org/10.1093/jncimonographs/lgu032

Lieberman, K., Le, H.-N., Perry, D. F., & Julian, M. (2024). Cultural adaptation and a pilot study of the mothers and babies course for perinatal African American adolescents. *Journal of Child and Family Studies, 33*(2), 473–486. https://doi.org/10.1007/s10826-023-02588-y

St. Lawrence, J. S., Brasfield, T. L., Jefferson, K. W., Alleyne, E., O'Bannon, R. E., III, & Shirley, A. (1995). Cognitive-behavioral intervention to reduce African American adolescents' risk for HIV infection. *Journal of Consulting and Clinical Psychology, 63*(2), 221–237. https://doi.org/10.1037/0022-006X.63.2.221

Webb, M., Beckstead, J., Meininger, J., & Robinson, S. (2006). Stress management for African American women with elevated blood pressure: A pilot study. *Biological Research for Nursing, 7*(3), 187–196. https://doi.org/10.1177/1099800405283144

Substance Use

El-Mohandes, A. A. E., El-Khorazaty, M. N., Kiely, M., & Gantz, M. G. (2011). Smoking cessation and relapse among pregnant African-American smokers in Washington, DC. *Maternal and Child Health Journal, 15*(Suppl 1), S96–S105. https://doi.org/10.1007/s10995-011-0825-6

El-Mohandes, A., Windsor, R., Tan, S., Perry, D., Gantz, M., & Kiely, M. (2013). A Randomized clinical trial of trans-dermal nicotine replacement in pregnant African-American smokers. *Maternal and Child Health Journal, 17*(5), 897–906. https://doi.org/10.1007/s10995-012-1069-9

Montgomery, L., Robinson, C., Seaman, E. L., & Haeny, A. M. (2017). A scoping review and meta-analysis of psychosocial and pharmacological treatments for cannabis and tobacco use among African Americans. *Psychology of Addictive Behaviors, 31*(8), 922–943. https://doi.org/10.1037/adb0000326

Webb, M. S., de Ybarra, D. R., & Baker, E. A. (2010). Cognitive-behavioral therapy to promote smoking cessation among African American Smokers: A randomized clinical trial. *Journal of Consulting and Clinical Psychology, 78*(1), 24–33. https://doi.org/10.1037/a0017669

Webb Hooper, M., Antoni, M. H., Okuyemi, K., Dietz, N. A., & Resnicow, K. (2017). Randomized controlled trial of group-based culturally specific cognitive behavioral therapy among African American Smokers. *Nicotine and Tobacco Research: Official Journal of the Society for Research on Nicotine and Tobacco, 19*(3), 333–341. https://doi.org/10.1093/ntr/ntw181

Therapeutic Communication

Bhui, K., Aslam, R. W., Palinski, A., McCabe, R., Johnson, M. R. D., Weich, S., Singh, S. P., Knapp, M., Ardino, V., & Szczepura, A. (2015). Interventions designed to improve therapeutic communications between black and minority ethnic people and professionals working in psychiatric services: a systematic review of the evidence for their effectiveness. *Health Technology Assessment (Winchester, England), 19*(31), vii. https://doi.org/10.3310/hta19310

Appendix B: Cognitive-Behavioral Principles for Black Americans: RESPPECTUS

Principle 1	**R**esilience and Strength of Black Americans	
	Function:	Resilience and Strength of Black Americans principle calls for cognitive-behavioral clinicians to collaboratively and systematically identify and use the resilience and strengths of Black American clients to accomplish their treatment goals and personal aspirations.
Principle 2	**E**mpathy for Black Traumatic Events and Stressors	
	Function:	This principle is manifested in verbal and non-verbal communicative behaviors that convey accurate and authentic understanding of Black American clients' perceptions and impacts of Black traumatic events and the structural forces which perpetuate them.
Principle 3	**S**tructural Racism—Influences on Presenting Problems, Rapport, and Therapy	
	Function:	If structural factors are identified as being meaningful contributors to the presenting problem and/or the development of beliefs, these issues should be specified in the cognitive-behavioral case formulation.
Principle 4	**P**roblem-Solving	
	Function:	Problem-solving in a fundamental intervention that is used to address those situations that are rooted in structural and interpersonal racism and not solely explained by errors in appraisal.
Principle 5	**P**olicy Change	
	Function:	The primary function of the Policy Change principle is the cognitive-behavioral clinician's understanding of and engagement in upstream-oriented activities to improve micro level functioning for Black American clients with mental illness and addiction.
Principle 6	**E**valuating Thoughts and Beliefs	
	Function:	The primary function of the Evaluating Thoughts and Beliefs principle involves cognitive restructuring in a collaborative, empathetic, and structurally informed manner, that makes constructive use of each Black client's individual and collective resilience and strength.
Principle 7	**C**ritical Evaluation of Clinical and other Relevant Research	
	Function:	Cognitive-behavioral clinicians must identify and critically evaluate the external validity, intersectionality, and overall utility of extant research literature for the Black American client(s) they are working with.

V. L. Gregory, Jr., *Cognitive-Behavioral Therapy with Black Americans*,
https://doi.org/10.1007/978-3-032-01666-9

Principle 8	Truth and Transparency	
	Function:	The principle of Truth and Transparency calls for the cognitive-behavioral clinician to proactively create a therapeutic culture of truth and transparency. This culture of Truth and Transparency includes not only the clinician and their interactions with clients, but also clinical supervisors and agency policy.
Principle 9	Uniqueness of Each Black Individual	
	Function:	The Uniqueness of Each Black Individual principle recognizes the within-group diversity among Black American clients and uses Black heterogeneity to inform their work with Black clients.
Principle 10	Social Support's Import	
	Function:	The primary function of the Social Support's Import principle is to promote cognitive-behavioral therapists in aiding Black American clients in engaging and sustaining social support networks that may be beneficial for addressing racial discrimination, various forms of psychological distress, and other stressors.

Appendix C: Cultural Trauma Scale: 27 Items, Five Factors

Factor 1:	**American and Its Justice System: Cognitive-Emotional Responses**
Item 1	I do not trust the American justice system
Item 2	America is against Black people
Item 3	The American justice system is designed to keep Black people down
Item 4	I am disappointed in how America treats Black people
Item 5	You're more likely to be found guilty if you are Black
Item 6	When police officers kill Black people, the justice system does not hold them accountable for their actions
Item 7	Seeing African Americans die by police actions has forever changed the way I view this country
Item 8	There should be more Black people working in the American justice system
Item 9	I am emotionally drained by the Black racial injustice in this country
Item 10	Seeing Black people being killed by police makes me want revenge
Factor 2:	**Cognitive-Behavioral Coping**
Item 11	Social media plays an important role in educating people about important Black social issues
Item 12	My community helps me deal with Black racial injustice
Item 13	Social media plays an important role in gaining support for protests
Item 14	My family relationships help me deal with Black racial injustice
Item 15	Black racial injustice issues have caused me to lose sleep
Item 16	Changing my thinking helps me cope with Black racial injustice issues
Item 17	Mental health services are a great way to cope with the effects of Black racial injustice
Factor 3:	**Willingness to Seek Treatment for Cultural Trauma**
Item 18	I am willing to discuss Black racial injustice issues with mental health professionals
Item 19	I am willing to discuss Black racial injustice issues with medical professionals
Factor 4:	**Tripartite Police Fear**
Item 20	I fear for my life due to Black racial injustice in America
Item 21	I fear for my family members' lives due to Black racial injustice in America

V. L. Gregory, Jr., *Cognitive-Behavioral Therapy with Black Americans*,
https://doi.org/10.1007/978-3-032-01666-9

Item 22	I get extremely nervous when I see police
Item 23	Black racial injustice causes my family members to worry about my safety
Factor 5:	**Resilience**
Item 24	Protests should always be peaceful and nonviolent
Item 25	God will give us the justice that we seek in America
Item 26	Something positive will come from all of these negative Black racial injustice issues
Item 27	Black racial injustice will not stop me from achieving my goals

Likert Responses: 1—Strongly Disagree, 2—Disagree, 3—Slightly Disagree, 4—Neither Agree Nor Disagree, 5—Slightly Agree, 6—Agree, 7—Strongly Agree; Gregory & Tucker Edmonds, 2024 (Used with permission of American Psychological Association, from Gregory, V. L., Jr., & Tucker Edmonds, J. L. (2024). Cultural Trauma Scale: Psychometric evaluation of Black men's beliefs, emotions, and coping. *Psychological Trauma: Theory, Research, Practice, and Policy*, 16(8), 1329–1337; permission conveyed through Copyright Clearance Center, Inc.)

Appendix D: Cultural Trauma Scale: 22 Items, Six Factors

Factor 1:	Tripartite Police Fear
Item 1	Black racial injustice issues have caused me to lose sleep
Item 2	I fear for my life due to Black racial injustice in America
Item 3	I get extremely nervous when I see police
Item 4	I fear for my family members' lives due to Black racial injustice in America
Item 5	Black racial injustice causes my family members to worry about my safety
Factor 2:	**Beliefs about American and Its Justice System**
Item 6	Black racial injustice will not stop me from achieving my goals
Item 7	The American justice system is designed to keep Black people down
Item 8	America is against Black people
Item 9	When police officers kill Black people, the justice system does not hold them accountable for their actions
Item 10	I do not trust the American justice system
Item 11	Seeing African Americans die by police actions has forever changed the way I view this country
Factor 3:	**Black Injustice Emotions**
Item 12	I am extremely upset by the killings of African Americans, by police.
Item 13	The American justice system needs to be completely reformed.
Item 14	I feel so sad when I see Black people being killed by police in America
Factor 4:	**Cognitive-Behavioral Coping**
Item 15	My friends help me cope with Black racial injustice
Item 16	My community helps me deal with Black racial injustice
Item 17	My family relationships help me deal with Black racial injustice
Factor 5:	**Willingness to Seek Cultural Trauma Treatment**
Item 18	I am willing to discuss Black racial injustice issues with medical professionals
Item 19	I am willing to discuss Black racial injustice issues with mental health professionals

V. L. Gregory, Jr., *Cognitive-Behavioral Therapy with Black Americans*, https://doi.org/10.1007/978-3-032-01666-9

Factor 6:	**Resilience**
Item 20	Protests should always be peaceful and nonviolent
Item 21	God will give us the justice that we seek in America
Item 22	Changing my thinking helps me cope with Black racial injustice issues

Likert Responses: 1—Strongly Disagree, 2—Disagree, 3—Slightly Disagree, 4—Neither Agree Nor Disagree, 5—Slightly Agree, 6—Agree, 7—Strongly Agree; Gregory & Tucker Edmonds, 2024 (Reproduced from Gregory, V. L., Jr., & Tucker Edmonds, J. L. (2024). Cultural Trauma Scale (CuTS): Parsimonious principal component analysis, independent Black American male sample. *Journal of Aggression, Maltreatment & Trauma*, 33(3), 369–386, Table 2. This table is derived in part from an article published in *Journal of Aggression, Maltreatment & Trauma* on 11th September 2023. © Taylor & Francis Ltd. Available online: https://www.tandfonline.com/doi/10.1080/10926771.2023.2256741; reprinted by permission of Informa UK Limited, trading as Taylor & Francis Ltd.)

Index

V. L. Gregory, Jr., *Cognitive-Behavioral Therapy with Black Americans*, https://doi.org/10.1007/978-3-032-01666-9

9783032016652